"Sal Di Stefano is brilliant and my go-to source for all things fitness. He bridges a crucial divide, presenting cutting edge fat-loss techniques while keeping in sight the science of living and aging well. We live in challenging times, and Sal expresses a true understanding of the hurdles real people must go through in order to see results today. Anyone who reads this book and follows Sal's advice will see improvements right away, both in mindset and in the mirror."

—MAX LUGAVERE, author of *Genius Foods* and *The Genius Life*

"You don't just read this book—you do it, and you get the body you've always wanted. It's never too late to get into great shape, so this is a must-read for anyone at any age who wants to lose fat, build muscle, and get strong . . . for life."

—MICHAEL MATTHEWS, bestselling fitness author and founder of Legion Athletics

THE RESISTANCE TRAINING REVOLUTION

Hachette Go, an imprint of Hachette Books
Hachette Book Group
1290 Avenue of the Americas
New York, NY 10104
HachetteGo.com
Facebook.com/HachetteGo
Instagram.com/HachetteGo

First Edition: April 2021

Hachette Books is a division of Hachette Book Group, Inc.

The Hachette Go and Hachette Books name and logos are trademarks of Hachette Book Group, Inc.

The publisher is not responsible for websites (or their content) that are not owned by the publisher.

Print book interior design by Trish Wilkinson

Library of Congress Cataloging-in-Publication Data has been applied for.

ISBNs: 978-0-306-92378-4 (hardcover); 978-0-306-92377-7 (ebook)

Library of Congress Control Number: 2021931707

Printed in the United States of America

LSC-C

Printing 1, 2021

This book is dedicated to all of the clients I trained
throughout the last two decades as a personal trainer.
Thank you for trusting me with your health and thank you for
allowing me to guide you on your fitness and health journey.

I'd also like to thank my beautiful wife, Jessica.
You've been my number one fan and supporter since day one.
Without you, this book would have never been possible.
You brought me out of my darkest times, and you showed
me how to love fully without fear. I love you.

And a special thanks to my brothers and partners in Mind Pump.
Adam, Justin, and Doug, your leadership, friendship, and
support drive me to be the best man I can be every single day.

CONTENTS

INTRODUCTION

I was shocked when I read this statistic from a recent large study: 60 percent of American adults are *not doing the one activity* that can most effectively save them from obesity, diabetes, osteoporosis, chronic pain, premature aging, depression, anxiety, and life-crushing illnesses. They are *not doing the one activity* that best assures them an attractive, fit body and a happy, healthful, and youthful life.

That one activity is resistance training, a system of muscle-strengthening exercises and techniques.

Why aren't people taking advantage of resistance training and all it offers? The researchers hit the nail on the head and drove it down deep with one big whack: resistance training has not been as widely promoted by health professionals as cardio exercise.

As a result, people are pounding away on pavements or treadmills, bouncing around in aerobics classes, taking tons of steps on stair climbers. Yet, they are not losing weight but are actually gaining it, along with sore joints, bad knees, fatigue, and other proven casualties of cardio.

Yes, this is all totally true. *Focusing on cardiovascular activity for fat loss is a fantastic way to fail at fat loss and other health goals.*

This is an important message that I will expand on in this book because I'm passionate about getting it across to everyone in the world.

The seeds of that passion were planted a long time ago when I was a skinny, painfully insecure teenager. At age fourteen, all this changed after I picked up my first weight. And I never stopped. I learned how to build strength and develop muscle, completely rein-venting myself, inside and out.

As a teen growing up in the '90s, the biggest source of my informa-tion on resistance training came from the bodybuilding magazines. I studied these sources carefully and applied their advice religiously to try to build a strong and fit physique. I took this information as truth because it was considered common knowledge in the publica-tions I was reading, and I never questioned it. *Common knowledge is information believed to be so true and accurate that no one ever considers challenging it.*

In my late teens, I walked into a local 24 Hour Fitness gym and ap-plied to be a personal trainer. I was hired and did pretty well. Then, at only age twenty, I was promoted to general manager with as many as forty employees working for me. A few years later, I opened a wellness and fitness facility that offered one-on-one training, massage therapy, nutritional counseling, hormone testing, and acupuncture.

The vast majority of the clients I have trained over the last twen-ty-three years were everyday average people who were not interested in building massive bulging muscles; rather, they wanted to get leaner, fitter, and more mobile, and wanted generally better overall health.

One day, a client asked me: "What percentage of the people you train achieve fitness success?"

"Most of them," I said.

To which she replied: "All of them got fit and healthy from then on? No one fell off?"

That conversation got me thinking. I could help get people into shape, but helping them stay in shape was a different story. Most of my past clients could not maintain good fitness. My training approach had been ineffective. I had failed as a trainer.

From that point forward, I began to question all the so-called com-mon knowledge I had previously believed to be true. Americans don't have a weight-loss problem. They collectively lose millions of pounds every year. They have a problem *staying* fit and healthy.

I was eventually forced to reconsider some of the advice I was giving and rethink my approach, so I started researching the veracity
of my old beliefs. I looked at everything I had taken for granted as
fact. Little by little, I peeled away the fitness facade to reveal real
fitness truths. I was shocked to discover just how incorrect my advice
had been.

I changed practically everything I had done in the past and instead took an entirely different approach, based on new and accurate
knowledge. I started training my clients far differently than I had in
the past. Once the results started to come in, I was blown away at
how well my clients (and myself) responded. People got fitter, leaner,
and stronger—and got there faster and more easily. And they stayed
fit and in great shape.

Fast-forward a few more years: I met Doug Egge, who became my
client. We formed a close friendship, and together we created the first
MAPS fitness program. This acronym stands for Muscular Adaptation Programming System. It uniquely addresses a huge problem exercisers face: what to do when the body gets adapted to workouts and
you stop getting results. Phased into mini-cycles, our MAPS online
training programs keep you in "progress mode" so that your body is always changing and adapting for the better. Very few fitness programs
do this adequately.

Thus, with MAPS, our intention has been to counter the failed
workout techniques that I had witnessed as entirely ineffective. To
date, these programs have helped tens of thousands of regular people
get into amazing shape—and do it efficiently with less work.

Our challenge has been to introduce these programs to the masses.
A few years later, Doug and I met Adam Schafer and Justin Andrews,
and we started our fitness media company, Mind Pump. Our goal
was—and still is—simple: bring quality fitness and health information to as many people as possible, with integrity and honesty. We
wanted to shift the direction of the fitness industry from an aesthetic,
insecurity-based industry to one based on self-love and self-care—and

with methods that truly worked, not just in the short term but forever. We knew this could be accomplished with fitness education through entertainment.

What evolved was our online radio show/podcast and website, mindpumpmedia.com. Both are dedicated to providing truthful fitness and health information. The podcast is sometimes raw, sometimes shocking—such as *Why Meal Plans Suck* or *How Group Training Ruined the Fitness Industry* or *Carnivore Versus Vegan*. Whatever the topic, our goal is to communicate applicable and effective fitness and health information in a way that is fun and easily digestible. We want people to learn the absolute most effective way to achieve their health and fitness goals, permanently. Today, we reach millions of listeners with our website and podcasts every single month.

With Mind Pump, we initiated a revolution. Revolutions are the great turning points in history. They are tumultuous and transformative events aimed at changing a nation, a region, or a culture—in some cases, even the world.

This is what we are doing in the fitness world—a revolution—and this book is an extension of that.

I want people to know that the fitness world is filled with charlatans and snake oil salespeople. They push the latest and greatest (and sometimes downright dangerous) workout programs, supplements, and faux science on the unsuspecting masses by preying on insecurities and false promises.

I also want everyone to know that cardio, though it has its place, is *the least valuable activity for our body*, considering the context of modern life with its processed food overload and obesity-prone environments. A few pages from now, you will totally understand why.

So—welcome to the revolution!

The Resistance Training Revolution emphasizes resistance training to boost your metabolism; build lean, strong, and healthy muscles that exude sex appeal; and achieve health benefits you cannot obtain from other forms of exercise. With just thirty to sixty minutes a day, two or three days a week, you can look and feel noticeably leaner, stronger, and more attractive—even younger—than ever before. The best is that the benefits are sustainable.

Let me clarify something right up front: This is *not* a bodybuilding book. This is *not* a book about becoming a bodybuilder (unless you want to). This is a book written to help the average person get a healthy, fit, lean, and strong body that is equipped to withstand the unique health challenges of modern life. This is a book that helps change the way you look and feel—forever.

It goes against the grain of most strength-training advice and gives you insider secrets that I have learned over twenty years of working in the fitness industry—secrets no one has told you about until now.

The "secrets" are real and honest information not generally shared by the mainstream fitness industry. And why not? It's partly because it is hard to sell ineffective workouts and bogus supplements without lying, and partly because real long-term success does not come from beating your body up in the gym or by starving yourself.

In *The Resistance Training Revolution*, you're going to gain information and learn techniques that most people will never know. Here's a brief rundown of what I have in store:

- A program for getting lean, defined, and strong as efficiently as possible without wasting ridiculous amounts of time working out, regardless of your age
- How to get maximum results in minimal time—so no more slogging away at endless, ineffective bouts of mind-numbing cardio, which is a great way to get nowhere!
- Effective home workouts so that you don't have to waste time in your busy schedule going to the gym
- The exact formula for nutrition that makes losing fat while sculpting your body a breeze and for the long term. You'll learn the secret of "intuitive eating" to get the body you want while enjoying a broad range of delicious foods. You will not feel starved, deprived, or that you're "on a diet."

- Raw fitness truths that will show you what works and what doesn't. You'll be shocked at how easy it is to build lean muscle and lose fat once you understand these truths, and once you train your body the right way.
- The newly discovered health benefits of resistance training in terms of heart health, bone strength, joint protection, and especially antiaging
- Inspirational strategies that help you make fitness a lifelong habit

This book is for everyone, too—beginners, intermediates, even advanced exercisers. I will meet you where you are with new information and techniques that will not only change your body but also the way you train.

There's more, and I can't wait for you to discover it. I can't wait for you to start getting compliments on how great you look. I can't wait for you to begin feeling healthy and energetic after we get started on this journey together. Losing fat, building lean muscle, and getting healthy isn't as complicated as the fitness industry wants you to believe. *The Resistance Training Revolution* is your way to get there.

It's time for a change. It's time for a new approach. It's time for a revolution. If you want to get in superior shape, do it in a healthful way, and stay that way for life, this is the book for you.

Welcome to the revolution!

—*Sal Di Stefano*

PART 1

THE METABOLIC
FAT-BURNING
SOLUTION

THE CARDIO CRAZE: WHY IT'S MAKING YOU FAT

You've just caught yourself reflected in your full-length mirror. What happened to that once-flat tummy that now hangs over your jeans? Or maybe your doctor said you need to shed some pounds and is worried about your ever-soaring blood sugar. Or perhaps someone snapped a photo of you recently, and it made you realize that maybe you let yourself go and should be doing something about it.

I'm no mind reader, but let me guess what you're probably thinking: *I need to do something about this!* So, you decide to lace up your athletic shoes and start walking or jogging, and go on a diet. Or maybe you're ready to pull out that treadmill that has been gathering dust in your basement.

All good, but time-out! Yes, it's great that you want to lose body fat and get in better shape. Good for you! I commend you. But slow down! The exercise choices you make now can determine whether you lose weight and get fit temporarily or forever.

Much of the motivation behind weight loss and fitness for many people comes from a place of hating their body and hating the way they look. And that is okay (for now!). But don't let those feelings drive you to make decisions that are not necessarily the best ones for getting in shape. So, if you're eyeing your treadmill or ready to do laps around your neighborhood, you are about to head down the wrong road—the road of *cardio exercise*—to get to your goals.

As I emphasized in the introduction: focusing on cardio activity for fat loss is a fantastic way to *fail* at fat loss. Before I explain the reason for my shocking statement, let's have a heart-to-heart talk about cardio exercise and why it does not work as well as you might think.

CARDIO EXPOSED

Cardio, also called aerobic exercise, is any form of repetitive body movement over a period of time that promotes the circulation of oxygen through your blood. *Aerobic* means "with oxygen." When you perform cardio exercise, you breathe faster, so you inhale more oxygen. Your heart beats harder too. This gives your heart a good workout. Your heart becomes more efficient at taking in oxygen and supplying it to every part of your body. Examples of cardio exercise are walking, jogging, swimming, cycling, rowing, and aerobic dance classes.

I bet a lot of people have told you, *"You must do cardio to lose weight."* This is untrue. The cardio–fat loss relationship is greatly misunderstood. In fact, cardio is absolutely the wrong form of exercise for fat loss, especially in the context of the modern lives we lead. Let me elaborate.

Up until twelve thousand years ago, all humans were hunter-gatherers. Their environment was busy and very active, and food was scarce. They moved a lot just to get even a few calories to sustain them.

Our ancient relatives had to walk miles to get water, find edible plants, and forage for seeds, berries, and other plant foods since agriculture had not yet been invented. They had to hunt for animals and eat their flesh for food and calories. After spearing an animal, they had to track or run it down until it collapsed from exhaustion.

You'd think they burned a lot of calories from walking, running, and being on the move, right? But this is not what happened. Their body became very efficient at using the few calories on which they survived; they took in just enough to support their high level of activity. Their body (and ours) learned how to burn fewer and fewer calories so as to survive off the few calories that they were able to catch or forage for.

Unlike that of our hunter-gatherer days, modern life is busy but very inactive, and food is everywhere. We mostly hunt and gather at the drive-thru. Cars and other vehicles have seeped into our culture to such a degree that if we could walk or bike somewhere, we don't. Social media and the rise of online shopping have made us even more immobile. We used to have to leave our home to go shopping or meet our friends, but now we do it all over a device while sitting on our couch. And, of course, watching TV for hours on end is a national pastime. Our sedentary environment encourages obesity, and the current obesity epidemic does not show any real signs of slowing down.

Very important: we are also surrounded by easily accessible and highly palatable foods—fast food, junk food, processed food, and sugar-laced food. Within a mile or two of your front door, you can probably grab a double cheeseburger with fries and a milkshake. At no time in human history has this ever been the case. In bygone days, food was hard to come by, and even harder to get. Prehistoric life meant prolonged stretches of near-starvation, surviving on much-needed reserves of fat tissue.

Nor was food ever this palatable. We now have foods that are combinations of flavors, textures, tastes, and aromas that literally hijack our body's natural system of satiety (which is the technical term for feeling full). Typically packaged in boxes, wrappers, and other containers, those same foods are also engineered to be addictive.

In fact, multiple studies in lab rats show that they can get hooked on junk food in the same way that they become addicted to heroin and other drugs of abuse. So, we have a lot of rodents running around craving bacon, Twinkies, and Tater Tots. I wish I was making this up, but I'm not.

Studies on humans are even more revealing. Research shows that people will naturally eat roughly 500 more calories every single day when their diet is high in processed, ultrapalatable foods.

Think about it this way: If I took 2,000 calories' worth of plain, white boiled potatoes—no salt, no butter, nothing—and I put them in front of you, and told you to eat it all in thirty minutes, it would be impossible. You'd gag, palate fatigue would kick in, and you'd wave your white napkin in surrender.

But if I served you the same potatoes, but fried, salted, and processed in the form of a bag of potato chips (that's four to five potatoes), I guarantee you'd be able to wolf down the whole bag—and maybe within ten minutes. I'm not picking on anyone. I've done something similar myself.

So, here we are—sedentary and exposed to food that is highly palatable and ready to grab, practically on every street corner. No wonder it's so easy to pack on pounds and even harder to take them off.

So, what is a body to do in this day and age?

The very best insurance against these modern-life factors is to protect yourself with a *faster metabolism*. But that won't happen unless you kiss your treadmill (and other cardio stuff) good-bye.

CARDIO SLOWS YOUR METABOLISM

Metabolism is the sum of all the chemical reactions in the body's cells that convert food into energy. Simply put, it is a food-to-fuel process. The body needs this fuel to do everything from moving to thinking to growing. When someone tells you, "I have a slow metabolism," what they are actually saying is that their body burns calories very slowly, and this is why it may be difficult for them to burn fat. This person's body burns fewer calories than other similarly built people do. In other words, they have an efficient calorie-burning body, not unlike a hybrid electric car. *Efficient* does not mean "good" or "positive"; it means that there is a slowdown in calorie-burning.

The fact that their body is very efficient with calories would have been an advantage in ancient times, when food was scarce. Remember, our ancestors needed lots of calories to hunt, gather, and move the tribe from place to place in search of new hunting grounds for food and survival. So, a metabolism that quickly reduced its energy needs was a good thing in hunter-gatherer days. Over time, the human body evolved to burn fewer calories—the result of thousands of years of evolution.

But in our modern, sedentary society where food is plentiful, tasty, and fattening, this is now a detriment. You don't want an efficient metabolism; you want a metabolism that burns a *lot* of calories, even if you just sit at your desk at work. Under these circumstances, an efficient, or slow metabolism is a disadvantage because it increases the propensity to store fat and all the negative side effects that come with that—obesity, type 2 diabetes, heart disease, and other casualties of an unhealthy lifestyle.

So, the challenge is to abstain from food rather than find it.

Exercise, if you choose the right type, can really fire up your metabolism so that you burn fat readily. But the one form of exercise that does *not* accelerate your metabolism is cardio.

Here's why:

First, when you do any form of exercise, it stresses the body. Cardio does this in ways that make you better at cardio. Sensing this stress, the body aims to become more resilient to this stress so it can better handle it next time around. This is why you get better at exercise when you are consistent.

When you first do cardiovascular activity, you breathe hard, your muscles burn, and the activity feels just plain difficult. But over time, the exercise gets easier, and your only option from that point forward is to continuously do more and more cardio. This is your body adapting to the stress.

Look at it this way: Imagine if gas were superexpensive, like $150 a gallon. Would sales of V8 trucks drop? Of course, they would. Instead you would see sales of superefficient cars go up, or people would use public transportation, or just walk. We would have to adapt our behavior to make up for having to buy expensive gas. This is similar to what happens when our body is forced to adapt.

Second, cardio sends a signal to the body. This signal says, "Become *good* at this activity." Getting good at cardio means using less energy while doing it. With cardio sending this signal, your body adapts by sparing calories and pares down its primary calorie-burning tissue, muscle. This is why long-distance runners have skinny, stick-like legs with very little muscle. The hours and hours of cardio are making their body more efficient at saving calories, by slowing down their metabolism.

As part of this adaptation, the metabolic rate slows down because metabolism-boosting muscle is being sacrificed. This makes fat loss harder.

Burning fat becomes far more challenging if the metabolic fire is weak. This would be like trying to burn wood for warmth without the flame. It won't happen.

Maybe you've experienced this yourself? You start jogging regularly to lose weight, and it works, at first. But then things slow down, and progress comes to a grinding stop. Frustrating, isn't it?

Your body is undergoing metabolic adaptation, in which it slows down its calorie burn by reducing muscle mass. In extreme cases, such as prisoners of war, individuals have been able to survive on only hundreds of calories a day, but they were left with a weak body devoid of muscle mass. You need to prevent this from happening, or you will have a slower metabolism, and losing fat will become much harder.

So, with cardio, your body thus becomes very efficient at storing *more* calories and it becomes better at burning *fewer* calories. At the same time, you are losing muscle and muscle promotes a faster metabolism. The bottom line is that tons of cardio erodes muscle and slows down your metabolism, making long-term fat loss very difficult.

WHAT HAPPENS WHEN YOUR METABOLISM SLOWS DOWN?

A couple of things. For starters, your body desperately holds onto fat. Years ago, I trained an experienced bikini competitor. Shelly came to me after her body started acting as if it did not belong to her anymore.

RAW FITNESS TRUTH #1

PHYSICALLY BURNING CALORIES IS NOT THE BEST WAY TO LOSE WEIGHT.

All our lives, we have been told that if we just moved more, we should be able to keep fat off our body. But this is not true. Activity alone is a terrible way to lose fat.

The most powerful proof of this fact comes from the Hadza tribe, hunter-gatherers in northern Tanzania. They have a highly active lifestyle, foraging for wild food and game all day and regularly covering long distances on foot. They are moving much of the time, typically in moderate and sustained activity—much like our version of cardio exercise—rather than in explosive bursts. Nor do they do heavy lifting. They needs lots of endurance to live their lives rather than lots of muscle or strength.

Their diet is natural, made up of meats, vegetables, and fruits, as well as lots of honey. In fact, they get 15 to 20 percent of their calories from honey, a simple carbohydrate.

A scientist named Herman Pontzer has been studying the Hadza for more than ten years. One of Pontzer's central research questions was whether the Hadza burned more calories than their inactive counterparts in industrialized societies. What he and his research team discovered was so mind-blowing that at first they thought they had made a mistake: despite their highly active lifestyle, the Hadza burn a similar amount of calories as city-dwelling Americans and Europeans. The metabolism of the Hadza had adapted and slowed down so that they could survive on only the few calories they ate daily.

Pontzer's findings underscore the fact that inactivity is *not* the source of modern obesity and that cardio-type exercise is an ineffective tool for weight loss. Obesity is a disease of overindulgence of energy imbalance—more food goes in than can be burned off, especially with a sluggish metabolism. Put another way: people

continues

continued

gain weight when the calories they eat exceed the calories they expend.

Even for highly trained people, physical activity accounts for only a small portion of their daily calorie burn. Most of that energy budget is spent behind the scenes on keeping cells, tissues, and organs in proper working order.

But don't quit your workouts just yet. Although the Hadza use up most of their total energy on being active, an inactive body is subject to disease-producing inflammation and a high sensitivity to stress, which can lead to illness. This compromised energy mechanism can be overturned by regular physical activity, which makes exercise essential for overall health. But in the words of Pontzer, "in order to end obesity, we need to fix our diet." He understands that we simply eat too much for how many calories our body actually burns.

She had done eight bikini competitions over the course of two years, almost winning a pro card in the process.

While prepping for her ninth show, her body stopped getting leaner and fat would not budge, regardless of what she did. In fact, she was gaining body fat, despite doing 90 to 120 minutes of cardio every day and following a very low-calorie diet that consisted of broccoli, lean chicken, and tilapia.

Shelly came to me in tears. "Sal, I don't know what the heck is going on! I can't exercise more, and I can't eat less. I'm afraid that if I do, I'll gain tons of weight. What should I do?"

Her metabolism had adapted and slowed down to a crawl. To "fix" her body, she had to do what many people feel is unthinkable: cut her cardio way down and start eating more.

That's exactly what we did. I changed her exercise program and placed a special emphasis on building strength. I slowly increased her food intake. Here's what happened: Shelly did gain weight, going from

130 to 134 pounds. But at 134, she looked smaller, tighter, and more sculpted than ever because she had put on more lean muscle weight, which is quite compact and denser than body fat.

I tell clients like Shelly: Stop trying to burn tons of calories with cardio. Instead, try to build metabolism-boosting muscle with the approach I will detail in the next chapter. You will learn how to exercise less, eat more, and boost your fat-burning to new levels of efficiency.

When your metabolism slows down and your body holds on to fat, you also look "soft" no matter how much weight you lose. Ask any good trainer who has worked in gyms for longer than a decade what a "cardio maniac" is. They will know exactly what you're talking about. A cardio maniac is a person who comes into the gym religiously to exercise on a piece of cardio equipment for an hour or more every day. They all look the same. They have very little muscle. They have a flabby body. None of them is lean. In fact, most of them have excess body fat.

What is going on?

Honestly, when weight loss is your goal, it's exciting to see the numbers on your scale start to drop. But shedding pounds does not necessarily mean your body will look the way you would like. I mean, you could cut your leg off, and you'd lose weight on the scale too. If cardio exercise is your main form of exercise, it can leave you with a soft-looking physique.

Your body composition—the ratio of fat to lean muscle tissue—determines your body shape. Ideally, you want to reduce body fat and increase muscle to improve your body composition. Cardio exercise, however, does the opposite—increases body fat and reduces muscle. This phenomenon indirectly increases body fat—which is why you will look soft.

In other words, all that work on the treadmill or elliptical might turn your body into a smaller but flabbier version of what it was before, instead of a tight, sculpted physique with very little body fat. Being soft and flabby is a major negative side effect of doing too much cardio exercise.

OTHER CARDIO CONCERNS NO ONE HAS TOLD YOU ABOUT

If your number one goal is fat loss—which it is for most men and women—and you are not an endurance athlete, cardio should *not* be the cornerstone of your workouts. I hope you get this.

Before we go any further, let me clarify something important: I am not saying you should never do cardio, and I am not trashing cardio. It does have its health benefits. In fact, a couple of thirty-minute sessions a week or some long walks are perfect for health. Cardio is one of the best workouts for building your cardiovascular strength (hence the name). It increases your lung capacity and helps normalize blood pressure. It floods your body with feel-good endorphins, relieving stress and making you feel great overall.

For these reasons, cardio is a useful form of exercise, but it should not be abused. At the risk of encouraging you to binge-watch Netflix on your couch, it's not the actual cardio exercise that is the big problem; rather, the amount people do. Inappropriate amounts of cardio, without proper strength building, can result in some pretty serious health conditions, in addition to creating a slow metabolism. Take a look:

Heart complications. Studies have been conducted, looking at the other end of the exercise spectrum, to see whether more exercise is always better. One of these studies was published November 2017 in the *Mayo Clinic Proceedings*.

Researchers found that people who exercised well over the national physical activity guidelines for many years were more likely to develop coronary artery calcification (CAC) by middle age. CAC, which is measured using CT scans, indicates that calcium-containing plaques are present in the arteries of the heart—a predictor of heart disease.

The study included almost 3,200 people. Researchers followed them for twenty-five years, starting when they were young adults. People who exercised three times the recommended amount—or the equivalent of 450 minutes a week of moderate cardio activity—had a 27 percent higher risk of developing CAC during the study period compared to those who exercised the least. Too much cardio over time is risky to your heart health!

Longevity issues. Exercise is supposed to promote longevity, right? Well, it depends. Studies have found that high doses of physical activity may do the opposite.

In one such study—the Copenhagen City Heart Study—moderate joggers (who jogged at an average pace three to four hours a week) had a threefold increased risk of dying early compared to light joggers (who performed light physical activity less than two and a half hours a week). For strenuous joggers, the risk of dying was nine times higher. (Strenuous joggers ran at 7 miles per hour on average, for more than four hours a week.)

The researchers concluded: "On the basis of current knowledge, if the goal is to decrease the risk of death and improve life expectancy, going for a leisurely jog a few times per week at a moderate pace is a good strategy. Higher doses of running are not only unnecessary but may also erode some of the remarkable longevity benefits conferred by lower doses of running."

Repetitive stress injuries. Over the past thirty-five years, the number of Americans who jog or run has risen twentyfold. In 2018, the number of US joggers and runners was estimated to be nearly sixty million. I'm glad that so many people are moving their body. But this activity can come at a price to your joints. Depending on what kind of cardio you do, your ankles, knees, hips, and lower back can take a real beating. Cycling can create poor posture in your shoulders and back. Even swimming, a form of cardio credited with being joint friendly, can cause shoulder issues over time.

These problems occur because cardio usually has a set type of movement that you do repetitively with no regard for balance. For example, running uses the legs and upper body in the same ways over and over again. To prevent overuse injuries, you need balance with your movements.

Low energy. Listen to your body for noticeable decreases in your energy levels. Your body cannot adequately recover from a demanding cardio program if you are simultaneously dealing with other stressors in your life. As a result, you get tired, worn-out, and prone to illness and injury.

As a rule of thumb, if exercise recharges your energy levels and makes you feel revitalized, then that's a sign that it's doing you good. But if you're overly exhausted afterward, it may be taxing your body and depleting vital energy reserves.

THERE IS A BETTER WAY TO LOSE BODY FAT, GET HEALTHY, AND FIGHT AGING

Given that cardio slows your metabolism, making fat gain easier and creating a soft body, and has health deficits, is there a better way to work out?

Absolutely. There is a superior method of exercising that just happens to be the only form of activity, according to research, that speeds up your metabolism and keeps you in a fat-burning state, plus improves your health and longevity. And you do not have to spend hours doing it; you can spend as little or as much time as your schedule allows. If you stick with it, in just several months, you can amplify your calorie burn by hundreds to thousands of calories a week, on average.

Imagine burning more calories automatically. Imagine having a faster metabolism. Imagine making your body resistant to gaining fat. Imagine eating more foods but getting leaner because your metabolism burned off those calories.

Sound like something you are ready to do?

Then, let's go. There's no better training method for fat loss than what you are about to learn.

2

DO WHAT YOU'RE NOT DOING TO BURN FAT

I f cardio is the absolute worst choice for losing body fat, what is the best type of exercise for long-term fat loss?

In simplest terms: whatever builds muscle. Muscles are very important, metabolically active tissue. This means they burn a lot of calories just to maintain themselves. If your body doesn't think it needs muscle, it gets rid of it and won't waste precious calories maintaining it.

When this happens, you're sending the following signal to your body: "Hey, body, my muscle tissue isn't useful." That is the *wrong* signal to send, by the way. Your body then responds, or adapts, to this signal by deconstructing that tissue—a loss that results in less muscle, more body fat, weak bones, and a generally flabby physique.

Your body will have as much muscle and strength as it deems necessary. If you do not give your body a reason to have strong muscles, you will lose muscular size, strength, and calorie burn.

If you have ever broken an arm or a leg and had to wear a cast, you were probably shocked at just how much muscle and strength were lost in a relatively short time. Muscle is expensive, and without sending the right signal, your body will reduce your muscle mass in an attempt to slow down your metabolism.

Fortunately, we know how to prevent and cure those conditions, and it has a name: *resistance training*, also called weight training, strength training, bodybuilding, or just lifting weights.

Don't let the fancy names throw you. Resistance training is simply working against a type of force that resists your movement. If it initially conjures up weight benches and barbells, you're right—partially. Sure, resistance training includes traditional weight lifting, but don't forget about dumbbells, resistance bands, even exercise using your own bodyweight. All it takes to count as "resistance training" is a force pushing back on the force you're generating, performed in a way that promotes strength gain.

When you do resistance training properly, you send the *right* signal to your body: build muscle and strength. For that to happen, two main adaptations need to occur. The first signal is central nervous system (CNS) adaptation.

The central nervous system consists of the brain and spinal cord. The brain is like a computer that regulates the body's duties, and the nervous system is like a network that relays messages to parts of the body.

Try this experiment: With one hand, take an object and squeeze it as hard as you can, except make sure the rest of your entire body is completely relaxed. This hard is to do at first because your natural instinct is to tense up the rest of your body, including your face. Now, repeat the squeeze, but this time squeeze your entire body along with your grip. You probably noticed that you were significantly stronger when you tensed up your entire body vs. when only your grip was activated.

This is due to the full-body activation of the CNS. As another analogy, think of your CNS as the amplifier of the body and your muscles as the speakers. You can have huge, powerful speakers, but with a small, weak amplifier, you won't get much sound coming out of the speakers. This is why it was hard for you to squeeze as hard as you could while keeping the rest of your body relaxed: your body naturally wanted to crank up your CNS for maximum effort. The way you'll learn to perform resistance training here will result in CNS strength adaptation. All exercise causes CNS adaptation, but what we want is a strength adaptation where the CNS learns to activate muscles with organized force. A good CNS strength signal feels strong, stable, safe, and powerful. A bad CNS strength signal feels shaky, unstable, and weak.

The second signal is that resistance training tells your muscle fibers to grow. Larger muscle fibers contract harder and produce more force. This is no big shock. We've known it for a very, very long time. And larger muscles use up more energy. They require more stored carbohydrates from muscles (glycogen). And they require nutrients and calories just to maintain themselves. Plus, bigger, stronger muscles burn more calories than smaller, weaker muscles do when you move.

So, with resistance training, the primary adaptation is getting stronger. The side effect of that is a metabolism that burns more calories—possibly as much as 500 calories a day!

For reference, it would take the average person roughly one hour of vigorous cardiovascular activity to burn 500 calories. Because most of us are too busy to try to manually burn 500 calories a day, doesn't it make sense to teach your body to *automatically* burn an extra 500 calories a day?

We absolutely can get everybody's metabolism to burn that many calories daily. In doing so, we could directly counter the problems that we have in our society—a sedentary lifestyle and the huge availability of overly processed foods.

Over the years, resistance training has been a stepchild in the exercise world, downgraded in popularity because cardiovascular activity has been so overhyped by health-care professionals, doctors, and even personal trainers. But with new and growing knowledge of its revolutionary benefits, it's time for resistance training to take center stage. It's time to make resistance training your priority fitness experience.

So, let's get down to business. I want to explain and clarify in detail what resistance training will do for your body, your health, and your life.

BURN FAT WITH A FASTER METABOLISM

Your body burns calories for basic functions: to support its tissues, organs, and physical activity. All of this adds up to your total daily calorie burn. The calories your body burns on its own, just to maintain itself, can be referred to as your base metabolic rate. We can boost this through building muscle and telling the body to prioritize strength, so that you don't have to physically move as much to burn more calories.

Calories are a unit of measurement that symbolize energy. Your body needs energy to live, and some people need more energy at rest than other people do. They have a faster metabolism. Burning more calories, even at rest, is a huge advantage because food in modern times is definitely not as scarce as it was in the earlier days of human history. With a faster metabolism, you can eat more without gaining body fat, move less, and stay lean. Sure, you could burn more calories by working out more, but wouldn't it be awesome to just burn more calories and more fat automatically? That's what resistance training does for you.

Muscle is a greedy tissue when it comes to expending calories (that's good), and it accounts for a huge percentage of your body's total calorie burn. The more muscle you have, the more calories you will expend and the more fat you will burn. That is what it means to have a faster metabolism.

Your muscles also burn more calories when they have a relatively consistent "get stronger" signal. This is why the "every pound of muscle burns X amount of calories" math can be off. I've had clients only add a few pounds of muscle to their body (which made them look more sculpted but not bigger), yet they were able to eat 500 more calories a day and still get leaner. With more muscle, their body got the message to prioritize strength.

The best way to make all that happen is to train with resistance.

This fact becomes even more important if you are cutting your calories in an effort to lose weight. Some studies show that almost half of the weight people lose through dieting alone is muscle weight, resulting in a *slower* metabolism.

Now these people have to eat even less—forever—if they want to maintain their lower weight. If you are like most people, you have been on a calorie-restricted diet. How hard was it to lose the weight by eating less? Could you eat that little forever to maintain your weight loss? Most people can't, which is why diets fail most of the time, especially over the long term.

Cutting calories without sending a signal to build muscle and strength will almost always result in muscle loss. Here is why: Your body is always adapting to its environment. When you cut calories, your body simply tries to burn less calories. An easy way to do this is to pare muscle down, especially when your body doesn't get any signals that tell it that it *needs* strong muscles. Dieting without resistance training kills muscle and slows down metabolism fast.

Plus, calorie-restricted diets sacrifice muscle for the sake of weight loss—a very bad deal. You lose weight but end up with a slow metabolism better suited for fat gain. Resistance training mitigates this by encouraging the body to preserve, and build, muscle.

You want to lose body fat, not muscle. As I pointed out in the previous chapter, when you want to shed body fat, what's the first thing you're told? Do more cardio. The solution, then, is to put in hours and hours of work on the treadmill, elliptical, or track, right? That is how you'll trim the fat, according to conventional advice.

Science advises something different, however. Plenty of studies have revealed that cardio is not effective for burning fat. They also tell us something most of us don't know—that there's a big-time disadvantage to doing hours of cardio: it will slow our metabolism.

Although cardio also uses your muscles, they are employed differently than when you lift weights or do strength-based resistance training. Cardio requires lots of endurance and little strength, and it manually burns lots of calories. Your body adapts by getting better at what it does often, so when you do lots of cardio, your body gets better at endurance and it attempts to become more efficient with calories so you can go longer with less energy. Combine this with the fact that cardio requires little strength from muscle, and you send a loud signal to your body that encourages muscle loss.

I'm a bit of a science geek who loves to study research papers. They help me, since I spend a lot of my waking hours telling people what they should and should not do, training-wise. One article that passed through my hands offered some eye-opening insights into the metabolism-building benefits of resistance training versus cardio.

The study was a comprehensive, statistical review that captured data from 392 participants and 270 controls (total 662 participants) across eighteen studies. The objective of the review was to see which exercise activity—resistance training or cardio training—had the biggest effect on metabolism.

The main findings were that (1) resistance exercise significantly increased metabolism in comparison to a control group as measured by indirect calorimetry (a calculation of calorie burn); (2) aerobic exercise and resistance exercise combined did not significantly increase metabolism in comparison to a control group; and (3) resistance exercise *alone* was the most effective for boosting metabolism; cardio exercise was not effective at all.

The message is clear: For a sustained, faster metabolism, resistance training is the best form of exercise. And remember, the faster your metabolism, the easier it is to burn fat.

SCULPT YOUR BODY

My favorite feature is the ability to use resistance training to literally shape and sculpt your body as you see fit. Here's a good way to look at it: Resistance training is to the body what Michelangelo was to a block of marble—artistry capable of sculpting a masterpiece—using the human body as marble. Back to cardio for a moment: Doing cardio only will give you a smaller version of your shapeless self. But if you're shaped like an apple or a pear now, after losing some weight—without resistance training—you will be just a smaller apple or a smaller pear.

With resistance training, you can place special emphasis on any part of your body and, like an actual sculptor, change how that part looks according to your aesthetic goals. No other form of exercise does this. If you like running a lot, you will use the same set of muscles most of the time. The same is true for swimming or yoga or Pilates or basketball—pretty much all other forms of exercise. With resistance training, you work all muscles and thus have *more* control over how your body looks.

And you can choose to work some areas more than others. Want more shape to your butt? Do more resistance training exercises for your glutes. Want more sculpted arms? Do more resistance training exercises for your arms. Because resistance training builds and shapes muscle, it gives you the ability to aesthetically change your look.

I have a couple of secrets in my trainer's bag of tricks to mold and shape your body with resistance training. They include selecting the most effective exercises, doing them in the right order, using the most effective rep ranges, applying the best frequency of how often you should train your muscles, and teaching your body to move better with less pain and stiffness through what I call correctional priming exercises. Once you apply these techniques, you'll get the great-looking abs, thighs, butt, or any body part that you want to reshape.

Resistance training will alter your body cosmetically faster than anything. So, if you want to change how you look, nothing will do that better than resistance training. It gives you the body you've always dreamed of having.

BUILD STRENGTH

This one is obvious. Most people know that resistance training is the best way to build strength. The secret lies in how it's done. When you apply resistance training, you are literally training to get stronger *every* time you work out. When you do other forms of exercise, your body does get stronger at first, but once you have reached the amount of strength needed to perform your activity, the body stops

RESISTANCE TRAINING VERSUS CARDIO	
RESISTANCE TRAINING	**CARDIO EXERCISE**
Metabolic Effects: ■ Builds a faster metabolism	Metabolic Effects: ■ Creates a slower metabolism
Fat-Burning: ■ Decreases body fat	Fat-Burning: ■ Increases body fat; can result in looking "skinny fat"*
Muscle Effects: ■ Muscle fiber size increases. ■ Muscle strength increases. ■ Many ways to challenge and activate all muscles and achieve progressive overload	Muscle Effects: ■ Muscle fiber size remains unchanged or decreases. ■ Muscle strength decreases. ■ No progressive overload, therefore fewer ways to challenge and activate all muscles
Bone Effects: ■ Builds bone density	Bone Effects: ■ Bone density is minimally improved.
Hormonal Effects: ■ Testosterone increases ■ Growth hormone (GH) increases	Hormonal Effects: ■ Testosterone stays the same or decreases. ■ GH decreases or is unchanged.
Functional Effects: ■ Improves mobility and flexibility ■ Strengthens tendons, ligaments, and joints ■ Helps with coordination	Functional Effects: ■ Negligible benefits ■ Can harm joints due to impact
Antiaging Effects: ■ Reverses many aspects of aging—prevents age-related bone and muscle loss ■ Increases antiaging hormones ■ Stimulates antiaging changes in cells	Antiaging Effects: ■ Negligible benefits on major aspects of aging ■ Overapplication causes an aging phenomenon known as oxidative stress, when disease-causing free radicals overwhelm the body's antioxidants and create tissue and organ damage.

*Cardio can increase body fat percentage due to muscle loss. If you weigh 100 pounds, and you have 20 pounds of body fat, then you have 20 percent body fat. If you lose 10 pounds of muscle but don't lose fat, you now have 22 percent fat (20 pounds of fat on 90 pounds of weight). If you lose 10 pounds of weight, but 5 pounds are fat and 5 pounds are muscle, your body fat percentage has stayed the same. Body fat percentage is important. A 200-pound man with 20 pounds of fat is very lean at 10 percent fat. By contrast, a 100-pound guy with 20 pounds of body fat has 20 percent fat. When it comes to health *and* looks, body fat percentage is what matters. Remember: Losing muscle slows your metabolism, making you look fatter or flabbier.

trying to get stronger. With resistance training, as soon as an exercise gets easy, you add more weight, or more resistance. You are therefore constantly challenging your muscles, and this keeps them in a strength-building mode.

STRENGTHEN BONES

Resistance training doesn't just build muscles, it also builds bones. This is a much-overlooked benefit of resistance training, especially if you consider the fact that a condition called osteopenia, which is the loss of bone mass and strength, affects almost twenty million Americans. It often leads to the bone-crippling disease, osteoporosis.

With resistance training, your bones respond the same way your muscles do—they get denser and stronger. That's because you're placing stress (resistance) on them. Like muscle, bone adapts to stress by becoming stronger. At the cellular level, bone cells start multiplying and producing more bone density (amount of bone mineral and a measurement of bone mass).

In addition, muscle contraction—the flexing and unflexing of your muscles—builds bone mass too. Muscles are largely attached to and anchored onto your bones. When your muscles contract, joints move, operating like the hinge on a door. The movement of the muscles and joints exerts a rotational force, or pull, on the bones, called torque. The greater the torque, the stronger the bones will get.

Resistance training is a superior form of exercise for bone building. Here is one of many pieces of proof: A study at the University of Arizona recruited women ages seventeen to thirty-eight. Some were bodybuilders; others were competitive runners; and still others were swimmers and recreational runners. For comparison, a control group was made up of women who did not exercise.

When analyzed by scans, the average bone density of the bodybuilders was considerably greater across the board than that of the runners, swimmers, and controls. This finding tells us that the bone-building effects of resistance training are clearly in a league of their own.

BRING HORMONES BACK INTO BALANCE

Hormones are messengers that regulate cell, tissue, and organ functions, affecting everything from stimulating fat burning to building muscle. Significant hormonal releases are triggered by the volume and intensity generated by resistance training. The primary hormones affected are growth hormone, testosterone, estrogen, and insulin.

Produced by your pituitary gland, growth hormone (GH) plays a key role in height, weight management, cellular repair, and metabolism. It is also involved in muscle growth, strength, and exercise performance. Levels tend to drop as we age.

You can naturally increase GH by training with intensity—a term that describes how strenuously you work out. One of the best ways to achieve intensity is with resistance training. Over the long term, resistance training optimizes your GH function, plus decreases your body fat. Losing body fat elevates your GH.

One of the fundamental hormones of the human body, testosterone is responsible for many functions. It helps build strength, is responsible for libido, and helps give us the drive we need to accomplish our goals. Although testosterone is known as the "male hormone," it is also an important hormone for women. Low testosterone among women can result in low sex drive, low energy, weight gain, and sleep disturbances. Appropriate levels of testosterone are thus essential for women's overall well-being.

If you're a guy, having low testosterone can be an absolute disaster, with effects ranging from muscle weakness to higher risk of heart disease, cancer, and depression. Usually, the higher your testosterone (within normal natural ranges), the better.

Although, when applied properly, most forms of exercise tend to raise testosterone in men with low testosterone, only resistance training raises testosterone in *all* men. It doesn't matter whether your testosterone is at normal ranges or even high; resistance training has been shown to raise testosterone across the board. But if a guy does tons and tons of cardio, his testosterone levels can plummet in the process.

**HOW DID RESISTANCE TRAINING
GET SO STEREOTYPED?**

Bodybuilder. Does this word ring any bells with you? What comes to mind? Arnold? Someone who leaves the gym only for body-building contests and protein powder? Muscle freaks? If so, blame it on stereotypes.

Many times when the non-weightlifting public sees a body-builder, all they can see are the insanely oversize, freaky-looking muscles. These images have been splashed all over the covers and content of bodybuilding magazines, creating a stereotype that people who lift weights will develop huge rippling and bulg-ing muscles. The truth is, these muscles were built by long work-outs and huge amounts of anabolic steroids and other dangerous muscle-building drugs.

But now, the norms are changing, helped along by the fact many pro bodybuilders have admitted to taking gobs of drugs to build their physiques, and so are the ways the bodybuilders are perceived. *Bodybuilder* does not always refer to a muscle head who is bulking up with tons of steroids. The reality is, whether you are working out to gain a few pounds of muscle or trying to lose weight to sculpt your physique, you are a bodybuilder too. In fact, you can be an ideal bodybuilder. This describes people who build their body naturally with resistance training, leading to a body that looks sculpted, tight, shaped, strong, and lean. Healthy and natural strong looks *good* and not bulky or unhealthy.

This is because cardio performed for long periods of time deteriorates muscle tissue and, in the process, decreases testosterone levels.

In women with low testosterone, resistance training brings their levels up too. But if you're a woman with testosterone in the normal range, it doesn't have a testosterone-raising effect. In fact, in my ex-perience, proper resistance training is a great hormone balancer in women; whereas in men, it predictably raises testosterone.

Whatever your sex, if you want optimal testosterone levels, you should definitely lift weights or use other forms of resistance training. This is because resistance training is *pro* active tissue while cardio is *anti* active tissue. Remember, the main signal resistance training sends is to build active tissue, and this requires balanced hormones. If your body is convinced it needs to build strength and muscle, it optimizes hormones to do so.

In women, an estrogen balance is key to fat loss, since an imbalance impacts the ability to burn fat as well as to develop and retain muscle. Enter resistance training, which regulates estrogen levels by increasing lean muscle mass, which builds metabolism and burns more fat. With my female clients, nothing balanced out their estrogen and progesterone nearly as effectively as appropriate resistance training.

Finally—insulin. This is an important hormone that controls many bodily processes. It acts mainly as an usher to carry blood sugar into cells to be burned for energy. It also signals the body to store fat under certain circumstances.

Sometimes excess blood sugar piles up in your system, often as a result of eating too many sugary, processed carbohydrates. When this happens, your pancreas churns out even more insulin to lower your blood sugar levels. This leads to high insulin levels in your blood. The cells then sometimes stop responding correctly to insulin. Over time, your cells stop recognizing insulin (known as insulin resistance), resulting in a rise in both insulin and blood sugar levels. More body fat is stored too.

Here's the cool part: there is a "magic formula" for stopping this internal chaos—resistance training. Because your muscles play an important role in utilizing blood sugar, resistance training makes those cells more sensitive, or receptive, to insulin. Cells open their doors to insulin, and blood sugar gains entry to provide energy. That dangerous buildup of insulin in the body is resolved—and it protects against one of the most common chronic illnesses, diabetes.

Diabetes affects more than thirty million Americans. It's one of the biggest causes of death in modern societies. Muscle mass and

RAW FITNESS TRUTH #2

RESISTANCE TRAINING SHOULD HAVE BEEN INVENTED FOR WOMEN.

The fitness industry has been plagued with more myths than ancient Greece. One of the most glaring is that women who weight train will look like Mr. Universe. There are still many women who are sidetracked by this common misperception, thereby avoiding weights altogether and bypassing the opportunity to achieve a beautiful, shapely body.

One of the biggest differences between men and women is their hormone levels and how these hormones behave—most specifically, testosterone. Testosterone bulks up muscle mass in most men. Men have significantly higher testosterone levels than women, and therefore increasing muscle mass for men is much easier. The vast majority of women cannot build huge, bulging muscles because they have a tiny fraction of the testosterone found in men.

There are so many benefits to resistance training for both men and women, but the some of the benefits are very specific to women's health. For women, the truth is that resistance training increases your metabolism so that you burn fat more easily (and women tend to carry more body fat than men), you build bone mass and prevent osteoporosis (which affects more women than men), and you balance your hormones (which tend to fluctuate wildly in women as they age).

Also, women who do resistance training feel a boost in self-esteem and gain renewed physical and mental strength because of their new sexy shape. Resistance training is a woman's best friend. I rest my case.

strength have a tremendous protective effect against diabetes, with one study showing a whopping 32 percent lower risk of type 2 diabetes when people have just moderate amounts of muscle mass. This effect was independent of other lifestyle factors, such as frequent drinking and smoking, as well as of obesity and high blood pressure—both of which are risk factors for diabetes.

HEALTHY SEX DRIVE

Resistance training is also great for sex. In fact, this was one of the effects that surprised my clients the most, especially my older ones. After about three months of training, they would usually bring the subject up in a slightly embarrassed way by asking me whether resistance training had any "other" benefits. I would smile and say, "Have you noticed an increase in libido?" To which they would usually reply, "*Yes*—is that normal?" Yes, it's very normal.

Testosterone is the main libido-driving hormone in men, and studies have consistently shown that resistance training has both a short- and long-term boosting effect on men's testosterone levels.

What about women? Studies show that resistance training has a positive effect on the "youth-promoting" growth hormone (GH) in women (and men). Although not directly a libido driver, low levels of GH have been connected to less energy and overall vitality.

So, to feel friskier in the bedroom, do resistance training in your gym.

BECOME MORE MOBILE

Mobility refers to your ability to move through full ranges of motion with complete control and stability. It is commonly believed that mobility is equivalent to flexibility. Nothing could be further from the truth. Only having flexibility, without stability and strength, dramatically increases risk of injury. Think of a baby. Babies have amazing flexibility, but they lack control and strength. This is why just getting flexible isn't enough; you also need to have strength and control throughout your fullest ranges of motion.

Although all forms of activity will improve your functional mobility over being sedentary, resistance training stands head and shoulders above them all. Most activities are limited and involve repeating similar movements over and over again. Example: Walking involves the legs in a very specific way and neglects the upper body and the core. It also is limited to forward movement with little twisting, bending over, rowing, pressing, backward movement, and squatting (just to name a few). All forms of exercise (besides resistance training) have this problem.

Proper resistance training involves full ranges of motion with resistance. You are encouraged to move in all kinds of different ways. When applied appropriately, you get stronger *and* more flexible. I can list hundreds of different exercises that can be used in a resistance training routine, each one of them strengthening the body in different ways. This results in a body that can move more freely with stability.

In the next chapter, you'll learn techniques to improve your mobility.

LESS PAIN

It's true that modern medicine has invented pills for everything, from flu to high blood pressure to diabetes, but the sad fact is there are still hundreds of ailments that cause doctors to simply sit back, scratch their heads, and say, "Hmmm. I have no idea what's wrong with you." Apparently, one of the biggest head-scratchers around is chronic pain. You hurt, but no one can figure out why, nor can they fix it. The typical solution to prescribe painkillers, which are not a long-term solution.

Here's the deal: much of the chronic pain in modern societies is not the result of an acute injury or overwork. It is a mainly a result of an immobile lifestyle. We sit at desks and look at computer screens. Our body molds to fit our chairs, with hip flexors getting tight, core muscles weakening, and other muscle-weakening adaptations. Truth: We don't hurt because we move too much; we hurt because we move too little.

Many people suffer from pain that comes from poor movement patterns due to weak muscles. Muscles move and control your joints. Your joints can move in optimal and suboptimal ways; properly strengthening the muscles that control them helps to ensure you move the right way. Allowing your body to become weak means your body has to compensate. You give the command to walk or sit or stand or run and your brain tells your body to move in the most efficient way possible. If a muscle is too weak to do its job properly, then other muscles will jump in. The result is poor movement and joints that suffer excessive wear and tear. You feel pain.

Resistance training is extremely versatile and can be molded to fit almost any person's needs. This is not true of other forms of exercise. You can specifically target movement patterns and muscles with resistance training, making it the best way to get your body to move well, regardless of your particular movement pattern issues. This is why physical therapists use resistance training almost exclusively with their patients.

Strong bodies are also less prone to injury. The stronger your back and supporting core muscles are, the less likely you are to suffer from low back pain. Getting strong the right way means you move better, and moving well means less pain. In the next chapter, I will share with you some surprising and natural ways to resolve chronic pain, particularly back pain.

ACHIEVE BETTER COGNITION AND MOOD

Another one of the most common comments I've heard from clients is how their workouts had positively influenced their mind. They felt sharper, could think faster, and were much more clearheaded.

Exercise in general has a profound positive effect on cognitive function. Working out increases levels of brain-derived neurotrophic factor (BDNF) in the brain. BDNF acts like a kind of brain "fertilizer," promoting the growth of brain tissue, and it helps preserve the health of your brain. High levels of BDNF have been connected with lower rates of cognitive decline and brain-related diseases, such as dementia, Alzheimer's disease, and even Parkinson's disease. Studies consistently connect physical activity with improved cognition.

Speaking of Alzheimer's, I've got some good news to insert here: Australian researchers have for the first time shown that resistance training can protect the parts of the brain vulnerable to this devastating disease.

The University of Sydney study, published in *Neuroimage: Clinical*, revealed that six months of resistance training slowed, and even halted, the degeneration in the hippocampus and its associated regions a year after the exercise trial.

The study involved one hundred people at high risk of Alzheimer's disease because they were showing a decline in memory and other thinking skills. They performed ninety minutes of supervised strength training (using dumbbells, weights, or machines) each week for six months. After the study, their cognitive deficits improved greatly. The senior researcher, Michael Valenzuela, said it was the first intervention that slowed or halted brain deterioration—and that it was clear that resistance training needed to be part of dementia reduction strategies! To date, *no other* form of exercise has been shown to do this.

Resistance training is particularly special in the brain-boosting department because of its benefits for proprioception; that is, your awareness of your body in space. Due to the thousands of resistance training exercises and the variations of each that are available, you can train your body in an almost infinite combination of directions, speeds, and ranges of motion. This trains your brain as much as it trains your muscles.

Whenever I'd get a new client, I'd have them fill out a health questionnaire. It probes about exercise history, daily physical activity, sleep quality, the presence of gut and digestive issues, diet (what they generally eat and drink), use of alcohol or drugs, and general health history questions. But it also asks whether the new client has ever been treated for depression or anxiety.

Those questions were very telling. I was always shocked to discover how many people have suffered from either or both of those ailments. Statistics verify this fact: 7 to 10 percent of Americans suffer from mild to moderate depression while surveys show that 40 percent of Americans are feeling more anxious now versus last year. Some professionals are saying we are in the middle of an anxiety and depression epidemic.

Exercise is a fantastic treatment for shaking the blahs. Studies comparing exercise to antidepressants show them to be at least equally effective at treating the symptoms of mild to moderate depression, with some professionals saying that exercise is a better long-term overall solution due to its wide-ranging health benefits.

Resistance training is one of the best forms of exercise for this kind of depression and anxiety because it forces people to be more present. Whereas you can get lost in thoughts or even think about stressful events while walking or running, you *must* stay present while lifting weights. Resistance training is not like other forms of exercise in which you do the same movements repeatedly over and over. Due to the high skill and high resistance, you must stay focused on your form and technique during resistance training. It is not just repetitive movement. Adding resistance training to your exercise routine can positively impact these important areas of your life.

REVERSE THE AGING PROCESS

Here's a no-brainer kind of question: Do you want to live longer and healthier or die younger and sicker? Doesn't take much time to think that one over, does it?

Let's start with the basics. Living longer better starts with not dying, and physical strength just happens to be an excellent predictor of longevity. Using data from the National Health and Nutrition Examination Survey, a team at Indiana University assessed 4,440 adults

EASE POSTPARTUM DEPRESSION WITH RESISTANCE TRAINING

During and after your pregnancy, many changes occur in your body, both mentally and physically. The birth of your child and the new role—of a mother—can sometimes bring on various negative emotions, such as uncertainty, fear, anxiety, depression, or sadness. After giving birth, many new moms develop the "baby blues," medically known as postpartum depression. It may affect both yours and your newborn's health. That is why it is so important to find natural factors that can ease this kind of depression. Fortunately, one factor stands head and shoulders above the rest: resistance training—for four reasons.

1. It saves time. Having a newborn is time-consuming! Life becomes even more hectic, especially if you have other children to take care of. You can barely carve out time for yourself.

Problem solved! Resistance training—as little as ninety minutes a week—helps you in a time crunch. Plus, it produces the best results in the least amount of time. Also, resistance training improves your metabolism so that your body learns to burn 300 to 500 calories daily, no matter what you do.

2. It solves joint pain. During pregnancy and afterward, back, hip, knee, and overall joint pain is common due to the release of a hormone called relaxin. This hormone loosens ligaments and improves overall flexibility to prepare for childbirth. After birth, relaxin drops back down to prepregnancy levels, but its side effects are still usually present. Combine this with the fact that your core muscles have just been stretched to their max and have shrunk and you have a perfect storm of looseness with weakness. The postpartum body then develops instability issues—the result of too much flexibility and lack of strength.

Doing flexibility-based exercise, such as yoga, postpartum may actually aggravate this situation. With the focus on flexibility, and a much lower focus on strength, it can further increase instability by making the ratio of looseness to strength worse.

continues

continued

Proper resistance training, with its focus on full and controlled ranges of motion, maintains flexibility, but it also builds strength and control within that flexibility. The ratio of looseness to strength improves and core, hips, back, and the rest of your body become more stable and stronger. The result: joint pain is resolved.

3. It sculpts your body. This unique ability of resistance training can quickly bring your body back to its prepregnancy fit shape—or better. It burns body fat—which is associated with depression. Not only does resistance training make you look better and burn fat, it also boosts your body image and lifts the anxiety associated with pregnancy weight gain. You feel better about yourself, and this eases postpartum depression too.

4. It balances your hormones. Resistance training releases dopamine and norepinephrine; both regulate emotions positively. It also boosts serotonin, along with endorphins; all of these are feel-good chemicals. Because resistance training tells the body to build lean tissue, growth hormone increases, the body's use of insulin improves, and the balance of estrogen and progesterone is restored. At the same time, cortisol, a stress hormone, drops. The net effect is to ease depression, and you feel better emotionally.

There you have it. If you just had a baby and are cleared for exercise, choose resistance training to see and feel the best results.

ages fifty or up who had their strength and muscle mass assessed between 1999 and 2002. The researchers checked back in 2011 to see who had died.

The results, published in the *Journal of Gerontology*, found that those with *weak* muscles (very little strength) were more than twice as likely to have died during the follow-up period than those with normal muscle strength. The stronger you are, the more likely you are to live longer. To delay death, lift weights!

Here's the deal: If you're over the age of thirty-five—and not doing resistance training—you've begun losing muscle, a process that will worsen if you don't take action. When you lose muscle with age, it becomes difficult to carry out such daily activities as climbing stairs or even getting up from your chair. This can lead to inactivity, which causes further muscle loss. You can therefore be at an increased risk of falling, a loss of independence, and even premature death.

Muscle aging is caused by several underlying factors—all of which can be reversed by resistance training:

- *Decreased numbers of muscle stem cells.* These cells are the only ones that can repair muscle, and they decline considerably with age. However, the number of muscle stem cells can be increased by exercise, and active elderly people have more of these cells than their more sedentary counterparts do, according to studies.
- *Mitochondrial dysfunction.* Mitochondria are the powerhouses of muscle cells. To work efficiently, skeletal muscle needs a sufficient number of fully functional mitochondria. A lack of exercise decreases the efficiency and number of mitochondria in skeletal muscle. Not good! But thankfully, resistance promotes mitochondrial health and function, so that you can continue to create new muscle.
- *Declining myokines.* Myokines are chemicals released by muscle cells to help muscle repair, recover, and grow. Resistance training can restore levels of myokines that decline with age—which means they can continue to help the body create new muscle tissue.

Aging is a bummer, but resistance training is truly the fountain of youth. It is the *only* form of exercise that can dramatically postpone, even reverse, the losses in muscle mass, bone density, and strength that were once considered preordained results of aging. Not only that, but resistance training simply makes you look younger with less body

DOES RESISTANCE TRAINING HELP YOUR HEART?

This is an excellent question. To improve heart health, conventional wisdom says we need to run, jog, bike, swim, or otherwise get our heart rate up—and the longer, the better, right? Isn't that why it's called "cardiovascular" exercise?

Again, science has a different take on conventional wisdom. Many studies show that resistance training can be a valuable addition in reducing the risk of heart disease. Here's how:

BETTER BLOOD PRESSURE

Research from Appalachian State University has found that resistance training significantly reduces blood pressure—in the short term and throughout the years of regular training,

LOWER CHOLESTEROL AND TRIGLYCERIDE LEVELS

Both are fatty substances that travel in the blood and can clog arteries, contributing to heart attacks and strokes. Writing in the *Journal of Applied Physiology* in 2013, researchers noted that resistance training can reduce the risk of both.

REDUCED FAT AROUND THE HEART

The body carries two types of fat. On the outside is subcutaneous fat—the kind we hate to see after putting on a swimsuit. Inside your body, around your trunk, is visceral fat, which pads your internal organs, including the heart. Too much subcutaneous fat can lead to ripping the seat of your pants the next time you go dancing. Too much visceral fat can lead to less embarrassing but frightening conditions, such as heart disease and type 2 diabetes.

People who are overweight tend to carry more visceral fat than people who are lean. Fortunately, resistance training can fight it. In a 2015 *Obesity* study of 10,500 men, those who resistance

continues

continued

trained for twenty minutes a day put on less visceral fat over a period of twelve years, compared to those who spent the same amount of time performing cardio exercise. That's powerfully positive news: not only can resistance training make you fit and trim on the outside, it can do the same on the inside.

SOUNDER SLEEP

Even the healthiest among us—those who eat right and exercise—often neglect a good night's sleep. If you suffer poor-quality sleep, heart health is one of the first things to go. Medical experts will tell you that sleep deprivation triggers inflammation that causes cellular damage to your cardiovascular system, plus increases visceral fat and insulin resistance (both risk factors for heart disease).

Research published in the *Journal of Strength and Conditioning Research* found that performing resistance training, especially in the evening, can significantly improve your sleep. That's what happened to people in the study. They slept better than those who skipped the weights. (I have additional strategies for better sleep in the next chapter.)

So, there you have it: resistance training is a great help to your cardiovascular system.

---

fat and more body-firming muscle. There is just no other bona fide age eraser than resistance training!

BONUS: IT DOESN'T TAKE AS MUCH TIME

An effective resistance training program involves only two to three days a week for only forty-five to sixty minutes each workout. Plus, most of the clients I trained did only resistance training two days a week.

This doesn't mean you shouldn't also try to be active on the other days, but this usually took the form of some daily walks or just generally being more aware of activity throughout the day versus needing to do a structured thirty to sixty minutes of vigorous cardio every single day. My clients were far more likely to be consistent with this behavioral approach.

For that small investment of time in resistance training, you will gain a significant amount of all of the benefits I listed in this chapter and more. This simply is not true of other forms of exercise, which yield minimal results.

When you combine the fact that you don't need to apply a lot of time to it and that it has been proven to give some of the best long-term benefits, resistance training should be the form of exercise you prioritize.

ONE MORE QUESTION: WHAT IF YOU ENJOY CARDIO? AND YOU WANT TO KEEP DOING IT?

No problem! There is a form of cardio I do recommend. First, some perspective: The traditional form of cardio is known as steady state (SS) cardio, in which you get on an elliptical or a treadmill and move at a continual consistent pace. This form is basic aerobic exercise because the main sources of energy used to fuel this type of cardio require a lot of oxygen and fat.

The other type of cardio is high-intensity interval training (HIIT). It involves explosive sprints of high-intensity work interrupted by short periods of rest. It is less aerobic than SS cardio and is more anaerobic, meaning that it uses less oxygen and more stored carbohydrates as its main energy source.

To contrast the two: If you run for long distances, you are doing SS cardio. If you sprint, you are doing HIIT cardio. You can see the differences between the two in the physiques they produce. Long-distance runners are skinny with little fat and little muscle, whereas sprinters are muscular with a lot of muscle and little fat. HIIT cardio is more like resistance training than SS cardio is.

In fact, when studies compare SS cardio to HIIT cardio, researchers find that HIIT may burn more body fat—even around your waist—and either builds more muscle or, at the least, preserves more muscle than SS cardio. This gives HIIT cardio a *huge* advantage, considering that one of the pitfalls of doing lots of SS cardio is a reduction in muscle mass and, consequently, a *slower* metabolic rate.

There are different ways to perform HIIT cardio. One easy way is to simply do short sprints on a cardio machine. For example, you could get on an elliptical and do 20-second bursts of maximal exertion followed by 40 to 60 seconds of slow, recovery-based cardio. HIIT cardio should not be done for as long as SS cardio either. A typical HIIT session should last no more than fifteen minutes—a real time-saver!

There is another method, and that is to combine it with resistance training, thus making your body even more efficient at burning fat. When you set up a HIIT session with resistance, you burn just as many calories as when you do HIIT on cardio, but you gain added benefits of some muscle and strength gain. This translates into a faster metabolism, which makes getting and staying lean much easier. You also get the body-sculpting effects that only resistance training can provide. I'll give you HIIT resistance workout on page 189.

A bit of a caveat: HIIT is very intense and explosive, plus a little riskier in terms of injury. If you've never done HIIT, I recommend performing SS cardio for a few weeks prior to graduating to HIIT.

I am confident that no matter what your goals are in health, performance, and life, resistance training will support them and push you along the way to achieving every single one. For its now and later payoffs, pick up a couple of dumbbells—please!

3

FORGOTTEN FACTORS FOR A GREAT BODY

How fit are you right now? Any aches and pains? Is your lifestyle healthy, or does it need some tweaking?

When I was training clients, I'd give them some simple fitness tests and assessments to see where they were starting from—and to gauge their progress later. I looked at several aspects of fitness that I call the "forgotten factors" in health and fitness: mobility, posture, strength, core stability, body fat distribution, and various lifestyle factors.

THE MOBILITY FACTOR

The most important of these factors is mobility, which I covered briefly in the previous chapter. Mobility in the context of physical fitness refers to your ability to move freely with control and stability. In other words, it is owning your body's movement.

I admit that the word *mobility* doesn't have the same ring or sexiness as other fitness-related terms. If I want to promote a fitness program, the best phrases I can use revolve around building muscle, burning body fat, faster metabolism, or body sculpting. Mobility doesn't sell fitness well, which is why most people don't know much about mobility or value it. This is too bad because mobility is really key to long-term fitness success, directly impacting both fat loss and muscle building.

When you correct and improve your mobility, you:

Stimulate Your Muscles to Get in Shape Faster

Mobility increases your range of motion—the distance and direction a joint can move to its full potential—when working out. Taking an exercise through a greater range of motion means you get more out of every rep.

Let's use the example of a squat. Suppose you add 3 inches to your squat depth, but the resistance you use stays the same. You actually build much more strength and develop more lean muscle from every squat repetition, even though the resistance stays the same. That's the power of mobility. You get more out of every exercise.

Move Better and Prevent Injury

Many people are naturally tight and immobile. This can drastically reduce performance while also increasing odds of sustaining an injury. Poor mobility is often the source of pain and injury, both in and out of the gym.

With poor mobility, some muscle groups tend to stop responding or doing their job as well as they should be when called upon. This forces other muscles that *shouldn't* be working as hard to take over, leading to pain and imbalances. Good mobility fixes this and improves how your body moves, looks, and feels.

Heal Chronic Pain

An astounding number of Americans suffer from pain daily. According to data from the National Health Interview Survey (NHIS), 11.2 percent of American adults (25.3 million people) have experienced some form of pain every day for the past three months. Much of this pain is due to acute causes, such as accidents, surgery, injuries, burns or cuts, or childbirth. *Acute pain* usually starts suddenly but doesn't last long. When you twist your ankle, for example, you suffer acute pain. Resting your ankle and staying off it usually resolves the pain. After acute pain goes away, you can go on with your life as usual.

A sizable percentage, however, is not due to an acute reason, but is the result of *chronic pain*. This type of pain is ongoing and generally lasts longer than six months. It is the result of poor mobility, problematic movement patterns, bad posture, tight muscles, lack of strength, and overall muscle weakness.

I compare chronic pain to what happens when your sliding glass door doesn't move right. It gets off the track by a little but will still open and close. But over time, the track gets chewed up by wear and tear. Its movement pattern is off, so the door no longer works optimally. The same thing happens to your body. When it doesn't move correctly, it, too, gets offtrack, and chronic pain is the result.

I've worked with clients who weren't even aware that they had chronic pain, usually because they had been on pain medications for so long, and they just lived with it. I'd ask all my clients whether they suffered any pain. Usually, they'd say no. But digging deeper, I'd get them to admit that, yes, they had low back, knee, or wrist pain that had bothered them for a long time.

The majority of chronic pain I've seen in clients was usually the result of poor mobility and muscle recruitment patterns. Either these patterns caused bad movement that set them up for injury, or these bad movement patterns created wear and tear in the spine or inflammation in the muscles of the back, which cause terrible daily or almost-daily pain. The good news is that pain due to poor movement patterns can typically be fixed in relatively short periods of time when the right types of correctional resistance training are introduced. Best of all, you can notice immediate relief.

Gain a Better Quality of Life

Better mobility means you're moving pain free, not just in the gym, but in your day-to-day life as well. You don't have trouble squatting to pick your kids' toys up off the floor, or reaching overhead to put something on the shelf. As you age, maintaining good mobility is key to being able to move and do what you want without restrictions.

In this chapter, you'll be taught how to incorporate mobility training for every single body part, from your hands down to your ankles. This leads to increased performance, less pain, better and more rapid muscle development, less injury, and overall better physique and posture.

You'll also learn how to assess the other fitness factors—all of which are vital to your progress.

For the mobility and other fitness tests, we will be doing the following:

POSTURE ANALYSIS

We spend most of our days hunched over a desk on a computer or, even more so, on our cell phone. Over time, our muscles adapt to this posture—which I refer to as "forward shoulders." The shoulders become rounded, and the head juts forward.

With this kind of alignment, the neck and shoulders are forced to adapt. They then get overworked, trying hard to support the weight. This is why you feel tension and strain in your neck, shoulders, and back—which then leads to headaches, stiff neck, and midback pain. Being slumped over all the time can also interfere with breathing and digestion.

Once you start a resistance training program, you can potentially put yourself at risk because you are now taking this bad posture and presumably putting it under a heavy load, which amplifies the risk of injury while also reinforcing the bad form. All of these side effects can kill your progress in the gym, and take away from your life outside it.

A posture assessment clues you into weak and tight muscles right away—and lets you take corrective measures, if needed.

The good news is that pain due to poor movement patterns can typically be fixed in relatively short periods of time when the right types of stretching and exercise are introduced. An unexpected bonus is the appearance of weight loss. Slumping can cause your tummy to jut out, which means that once you improve your posture, it often looks as though you've instantly lost 5 pounds.

The Test:

Stand barefoot and relaxed, preferably wearing a swimsuit. Have a trusted person take your picture from the back, the front, and the side—basically your whole body.

Compare your pictures to the following diagrams, which show proper posture.

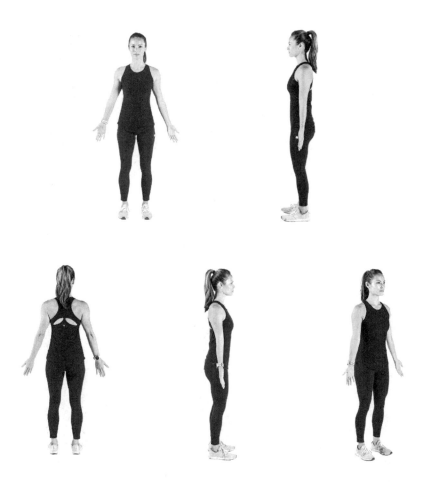

What to Look For:

Are your shoulders rounded forward?

Is your head jutting forward?

Does your lower back arch excessively to the point that your butt sticks out?

Is your tailbone tucked in?

Are there any differences between your right and left shoulder height?

If you said yes to any of these, your posture may indicate tight and/ or weak muscles that are causing distortions to your posture.

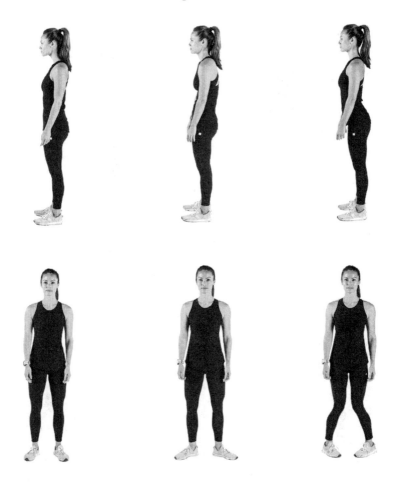

Also, keep these pictures handy. In four weeks, have them retaken. Compare the photos to your originals. You should see some amazingly positive changes in your posture—more well-defined muscle and much less body fat. Taking clear digital photos of the body on a regular basis is my favorite way of measuring progress.

SHOULDER MOBILITY TEST

In both men and women, certain crossover traits are universally considered aesthetic (that is, pleasing to the eye). There are many. Relatively lean body fat levels are one among them. Another one is the appearance of well-developed and sculpted shoulders.

Shoulders are the most prized body part of both sexes. Wider, sculpted shoulders make your waist look smaller, balance out your proportions, and help you look strong, fit, and confident. The shoulder muscles (often referred to as the delts) are one of the few muscles that both male and female clients will tell me they want to build for better aesthetics.

That said, the delts can be one of the hardest muscle groups to develop in the upper body. Their biomechanical actions in the body are poorly understood by many, and popular shoulder exercises are performed in ineffective ways. On top of this, people tend to choose the least effective exercises when they train their shoulders. (I'll correct all those issues for you in this book.)

The muscles of the shoulders enable the shoulder joint to move through a wide range of motion, making it one of the most mobile joints of the human body. Due to the extreme mobility of the shoulder joint and the muscles that operate the shoulder joint, it's no wonder the shoulder is one of the most injured areas of the human body. It's also another big reason that some people have such a hard time developing their shoulders.

The key to developing this valued focal point is mobility. Remember, mobility in the context of physical fitness refers to your ability to move freely with control and stability. In other words, it's owning your body's movement. Improving your mobility means you have improved your ability to move with control with larger ranges of motion. Working on mobility will make all the exercises you do more effective. So, in this test, we will evaluate your shoulder mobility.

The Test:

Lie on your back on the floor or an exercise mat. Make sure the back of your head, shoulders, and tailbone are pressed against the floor.

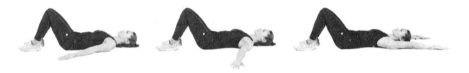

With your palms up, bring your arms up to about shoulder level. Keep your arms straight and bring them up, palms facing toward the ceiling, as pictured. Keep your elbows and hands against the floor, trying not to let them come forward. Any break in contact with the floor may indicate a weakness or area of immobility or inflexibility.

If your shoulders are very tight, I recommend performing this exercise daily or as often as you can. Try to increase the number of times you do the sequence. In no time at all, you'll see your shoulder mobility improve—and the shoulder exercises you do will pay off in the aesthetic look you desire.

THE SQUAT TEST

This test is a great way to assess your mobility, strength, and flexibility. It also mimics the movement we perform every time we sit up and stand up. This test specifically measures hamstring, quad, glute, lower back, and core strength. You will want to have someone photograph you from the front and the sides as you perform this test.

The Test:

Stand with your feet shoulder-width apart, and your arms straight up in the air, as illustrated.

Bend your knees, keeping your feet pointed forward, without any rotation of your feet. Go as low as you comfortably can—ideally past the point at which your thighs are parallel to the floor. Keep your weight on your heels.

From the bottom of the movement, drive back upward to the vertical starting position, raising your hips and shoulders at the same rate of speed.

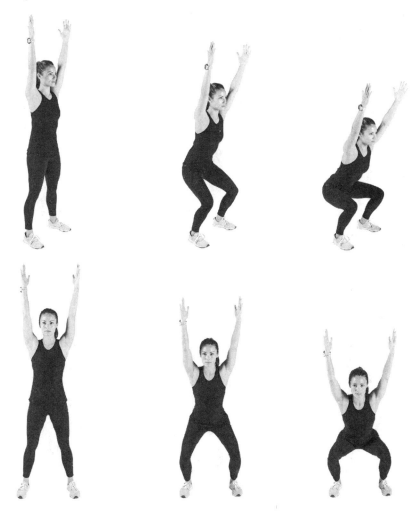

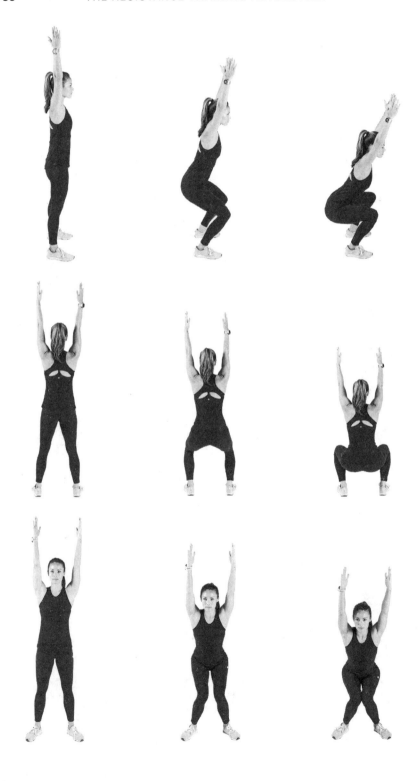

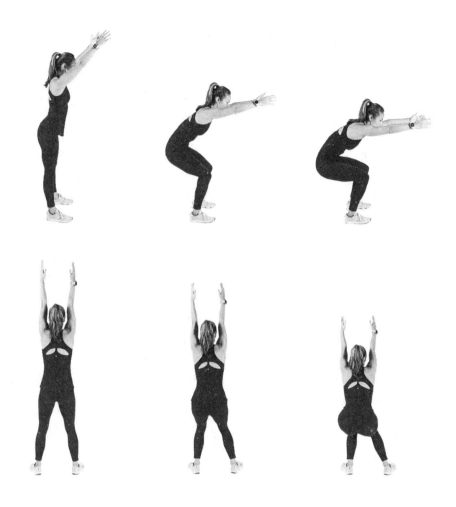

What to look for:

Compare your photographs to the photos here.

Are your knees collapsing, moving out, or not staying aligned with your toes?

Did your heels lift off the floor?

Did you round your back during the movement?

If you answered yes to any of these questions, this indicates a need to work on mobility and stability; inflexibility in your hips and a weak core; or weak glute (hip) muscles.

CORE STRENGTH TEST

Your core is like a corset. It connects your upper and lower body together and consists of many important muscles for human performance and function. The core is also an area that people will look at when determining whether someone is "in shape."

Visibly amazing looking and well-functioning core muscles are quite rare, even among fitness enthusiasts. This is partially because a visible six-pack also requires a low body fat percentage. If you aren't lean, it doesn't matter how well developed your core muscles are because no one will be able to see them. The other reason impressive core muscles are rare is that people don't focus on the right exercises and movements.

Having a stable core is a must to prevent back pain. When you can properly activate the muscles around the spine, much less stress is put on the actual spine itself. A stable core also keeps the spine in the safest position possible when loaded with heavy resistance.

Here's a simple test using an exercise called the plank that will help you evaluate your core strength.

The Plank Test:

For this test, you'll perform the *kneeling plank*. It is one of the best core-strengthening and core-stabilizing exercises around. It helps keep your back healthy, your posture tall, and your tummy flat.

The kneeling plank is an isometric exercise, meaning no movement is involved. Your muscles are tensed and fighting against gravity to stay tight. And while you may not be moving, it is definitely working.

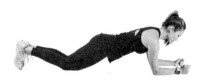

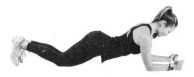 

Breakdown in form.

Begin by kneeling on the floor with your forearms on the floor, your elbows directly below your shoulders, and your knees on an exercise mat at an angle behind you. Your hips should not be sticking up into the air; rather, they should be tucked down so that your body is slanted but straight. Keep your spine straight, squeeze your glute muscles, and tighten your abdominal muscles as you hold the position.

Using a timer, see how long you can hold the position. If you can't get into this position or if you can't comfortably hold this position properly for longer than 30 seconds, you likely have some core stability and core weakness issues.

RAW FITNESS TRUTH #3

**APPROXIMATELY 80 PERCENT
OF OUR POPULATION SUFFERS LOW BACK PAIN.**

Ouch. What gives? Low back pain was one of the most common pain complaints I'd hear as a trainer. When your back hurts, you feel like you can't do anything at all. That's the bad news; now, here is the good news: through my decades of professional personal training, I have identified three main common reasons that there is so much lower back pain—and what to do about them. Number 3 might surprise you.

Reason #1: Overactive Hip Flexors and Weak Core Muscles

The hip flexors are a group of muscles that work together to bring your knee toward your chest and to bend at the waist. In today's

continues

continued

society, it is incredibly common to see people with tight hip flexors. This is likely due to the fact that we sit for most of the day and thus compromise our mobility. In a seated position, our hip flexors are shortened, and due to the length of time they stay in this shortened position, they tend to get tight. Combine this with a lack of core strength, and you have a recipe for back pain. If this is you, the solution is *not* to go do a bunch of sit-ups. This will only aggravate the problem and worsen back pain.

Also, when your core is weak, other muscles need to step in and take over. Often, it's the psoas, which can then get tight and inflamed over time.

The psoas is the biggest and strongest muscle of the hip flexor. It attaches from the lumbar vertebrae to the femur (from your spine to your leg bone). A tight psoas will constantly pull forward on your spine, sometimes making your pelvis stick out (think of a swayback-type posture) and causing pain where the psoas attaches to the lower spine. This needs to be taken care of right away, and I have the right exercise to correct it.

This exercise will get your hip flexors working independently of your core muscles and therefore correct "hip flexor dominance." This situation occurs when you do a core exercise, but your hip flexors are doing all the work. Or your hip flexors are tight all the time because you have a weak core. This problem is an issue for a lot of people, and it causes back pain or poor development in the midsection, so the movement you will learn here is excellent for improving mobility, alleviating back pain, and connecting to your core muscles so that your ab muscles develop much faster. You can eventually train your core properly for more rapid results.

Lie on your back on the floor or an exercise mat. Elevate your heels on a stable bench, chair, or even your couch. Your knees will be bent, and your thighs perpendicular to the floor. This position takes your hip flexors out of the movement.

This exercise also takes advantage of "reciprocal inhibition." This occurs when muscles on one side of a joint relax to accom-

continues

continued

modate contraction on the other side of that joint. In this case by activating the glutes, the psoas naturally "deactivates." Now, you can work the muscles of the core without working the psoas.

Push your heels into the bench or whatever sturdy prop you're using, and squeeze your butt muscles (this automatically relaxes your hip flexors). This is the beginning of the exercise.

Hover your back slightly off the floor. Tense your upper thighs inward toward each other slightly to prevent them from opening. Extend your arms out in front of you, and crunch upward as far as you can for a count of 2 seconds. Squeeze your abdominal muscles at the top of the movement for 2 seconds. Keep your glutes tensed. Lower back down to the floor in a count of 2 seconds. Breathe naturally throughout the movement. Repeat the exercise several times. You should feel your abs and glutes feeling tired—an indication that you are doing the move correctly.

Reason #2: Tight Hips

Anytime someone comes to me with back pain, I can almost always count on the fact that they will also have tight hips. When hips are tight, the lower back has to compensate because everything is connected. Loosening up those hips with flexibility exercises allows the hip joints to move more freely so that the lower back doesn't have to compensate so much.

An easy way to do this is with the seated leg crossover hip stretch, which can be done anywhere. In fact, I recommend that you do it every 30 minutes while sitting at your desk. You'll be surprised at how well this works.

Sit upright in your chair with your back straight, and cross your right ankle over your left knee. Flex your right ankle. You should feel a nice stretch in your right glute and outer hip. If you don't, slowly bend forward at your waist. Hold for 20 to 30 seconds, then switch legs.

Also, don't stay in one position for too long. Our body was not meant to be in a fixed position for hours at a time; it was meant

continues

continued

to move. Movement promotes blood flow, reduces inflammation, and allows muscles to stretch and contract. *Any* position held for hours a day can result in pain. Every hour you are sitting, try getting up and moving for 5 minutes. Walk, move, and lightly twist. This simple, mobility-improving tip produces amazing pain-relieving results for my clients. The side effects also include better cognitive function and work performance.

Reason #3: An Inflammatory Diet

A diet high in pro-inflammatory foods tends to make susceptible joints and areas of the body hurt. Pro-inflammatory foods include those that people are commonly intolerant to. A food intolerance occurs when a food is poorly digested or when your body has a low-level immune response to the food. Both of these cause inflammation in the body to rise up a bit.

Gut inflammation is caused by many offenders: eating junk food, drinking too much alcohol, being chronically stressed, sleeping poorly, taking too many anti-inflammatory medicines, such as aspirin, to name just a few.

Under normal conditions, the gut is very smart. Like a hall monitor, it permits food particles to pass through at appropriate times and places. But when the gut is inflamed, it can become "leaky"—a disorder called leaky gut syndrome, or its technical term, intestinal hyperpermeability, whereby undigested food particles pass through the intestinal lining when they aren't supposed to. The body identifies these particles as foreign invaders and mounts an immune defense against them, leading to systemic inflammation throughout the body. As a result, you develop an intolerance to certain foods, even if you've eaten most of them all your life. Symptoms of a food intolerance include digestive problems, skin flare-ups, brain fog, and poor sleep quality, among others.

Because intolerances are an immune system reaction or they cause such reactions, your body increases its inflammatory markers

continues

continued

to mount up a defense. This pro-inflamed state makes everything feel stiffer and makes areas that are susceptible to pain hurt more.

Many of the common offenders are otherwise perfectly healthy, but if you have an intolerance to them, they are not good for *your* body. They include gluten, dairy, eggs, corn, soy, processed sugar, alcohol, and processed vegetable oils, such as canola and corn oil. Overeating can also increase systemic inflammation, so try to eat less as well.

I'm always surprised at how many people actually eliminate most of their pain from these dietary changes alone.

BODY FAT DISTRIBUTION TEST

A body with more muscle and less fat keeps your metabolism charged up, but it also makes you look better. Most people—men and women—know this. But often, I've had women come to me and say, "I just want to lose weight." At that point, I'd ask one of my female trainers to come into my office. One of these trainers was Jennifer, who at five foot was very lean and in excellent shape.

"How much do you think Jennifer weighs?" I'd ask the new client.

The client said, "About one hundred or one hundred and five pounds."

I then invited Jennifer to step on the scale. To the client's shock, Jennifer weighed 135 pounds—most of it well-defined muscle, most of it sculpted and tight. I added that Jennifer can eat 2,500 calories a day because her muscle is expending most of those calories. The client could not believe how small and sculpted Jennifer was.

This type of demonstration was always a powerful way of showing how dense muscle is—and what building lean muscle does for a person's physique. Because of the remarkable changes resistance training makes in your body, I encourage you to do a body fat distribution test before you begin the program, and four to six weeks after. It's very easy to do and takes only minutes.

The Test:

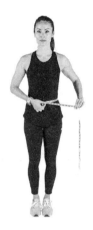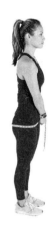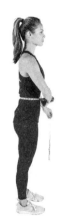

How to measure your waist-to-hip ratio: Using a cloth tape measure, measure your waist—which is usually 2 to 3 inches above your navel.

Then, measure the circumference of your hips at your hip bones.

Divide the waist number by the circumference at your hip bones. This math yields your waist-to-hip ratio.

What your results mean: The following table provides general guidelines for excellent to extreme levels for waist-to-hip ratios.

Also, take your waist-to-hip ratio every few weeks and watch it move toward excellent—which also means you're losing body fat in important places.

	EXCELLENT	GOOD	AVERAGE	HIGH	EXTREME
Male	<0.85	0.85–0.90	0.90–0.95	0.95–1.00	>1.00
Female	<0.75	0.75–0.80	0.80–0.85	0.85–0.90	>0.90

LIFESTYLE AND HEALTH EVALUATIONS

Apart from working out and eating properly, the way you live has everything to do with how successful you'll be at your fitness goals. I'm talking about sleep, gut health, stress, and attitude. All four require a reality check to see where you are and where you need to improve to arrive at your health and fitness destination. Let's start with sleep.

Sleep Assessment

Lack of sleep will kill your fat-loss dreams. When you don't get enough sleep, you lose significantly less fat than you would if you were well rested, even if the calories are the same. Research has found that this can make up to a 50 percent difference, so if you have 100 pounds of fat to lose, it could take you twice as long if you aren't sleeping enough.

One reason is that too little sleep leads to increased levels of cortisol, a.k.a. the "stress hormone." Chronically high cortisol levels have lots of negative effects on your body.

Notably for fat loss, when cortisol floods your system, ghrelin—the "hunger hormone"—is released with it. Ghrelin in turn stimulates your appetite. (The cortisol-ghrelin relationship is also part of why you want to eat when you're stressed out.)

Undersleeping also means your training sessions will be harder to recover from and will make it harder to hold on to as much muscle as you lose weight.

When you don't sleep enough: you're hungrier, you're more stressed, you have trouble building muscle and recovering, and you have less energy to devote to your life.

To Test:

Read the following statements and answer yes or no to each.

1. **I find it difficult to fall asleep at bedtime.**
   Yes or No

2. I usually don't remember my dreams.
   Yes or No
3. I wake up feeling stiff and achy.
   Yes or No
4. After waking up, I do not feel rested.
   Yes or No
5. I wake up earlier in the morning than I would like to.
   Yes or No
6. I am often sleepy and groggy throughout the day.
   Yes or No
7. I often wake up in the middle of the night.
   Yes or No
8. My mind races at night, preventing me from falling asleep.
   Yes or No

Scoring

If you answered yes to three or more of these statements, then likely you aren't getting enough sleep or good-quality sleep. See the suggestions that follow.

Gut Health Assessment

Your gut is full of three to five hundred different kinds of bacteria. They are collectively called your gut microbiome. Your microbiome is like a fingerprint, unique to each individual. But unlike a fingerprint, which you are stuck with for life, your gut bacteria can change throughout the day, based on what you eat, your stress levels, your exercise, and many other factors.

Many people are under the impression that the only symptoms of gut issues are digestive issues—bloating, cramping, diarrhea, nausea, gas, and so forth. But this is not entirely correct. Digestive issues are certainly an indicator of gut issues, but they are not the only indicator. Poor gut health can impact many different systems of the body:

HOW TO SLEEP LIKE A BABY FOR
7 TO 8 HOURS A NIGHT

Sleep is among the most healing actions you can do for yourself. There is literally nothing that you can do that will repair your body, bring hormones back into balance, and recover, like good-quality sleep. Although many of us need more sleep (7 to 9 hours is ideal for most), *quality* is just as important. I give my clients the following sleep routine, and it has produced great success:

- *Turn off all electronics one hour before bed.* The blue light from electronics reduces your brain's ability to produce melatonin and it keeps cortisol elevated.
- *Sip on warm chamomile tea.* Chamomile is a very safe and mild sedative and is even recommended for children in some European countries.
- *Belly breathe or meditate for 3 minutes before bed.* Belly breathing helps bring a calming response in the body, which is necessary for quality sleep.

To do belly breathing: Lie on your back. Place one hand on your upper chest and another on your belly. Take a deep breath into your belly and make the hand that is on your belly rise fully *before* the hand on your chest rises. This technique allows for a full diaphragmatic breath that signals the body to relax.

- *Do resistance training.* It has been scientifically validated to improve sleep. But perform your workouts earlier in the day and not so close to bedtime.
- *Create the right sleep environment.* Your bedroom should be dark, with a cool temperature. Both conditions are conducive to quality sleep.
- *Set up a consistent sleep schedule and stick to it, even on weekends.* Get up at around the same time each morning, and go to bed at the same time in the evening.

Your weight: Your gut influences craving and eating patterns. Some types of bacterial can increase your appetite for sugar or fats, or just make you want to eat more.

One study showed that lean people have 70 percent more diversity in gut bacteria than do those who are overweight. There are also certain bacteria strains that can cause the body to ultimately store more or less fat.

The immune system: Seventy to 80 percent of your immune system resides in your gut. The gut is where your immune system's T cells develop. T cells are a type of white blood cell that focuses on foreign substances that invade the body. It is in the gut where the T cells learn the difference between a foreign substance and your body's own tissues.

Your mental health: According to the most recent research, it appears that the gut is almost like a second brain because, like our brain, it is composed of a complex network of neural tissue called neurons. Our "second brain" can function independently and in coordination with the central nervous system. It is called the enteric nervous system (ENS).

The ENS can perform some duties independent of the brain, such as coordinating reflexes and secreting enzymes, one of which is the mood-regulating brain chemical serotonin. In fact, your gut produces about 95 percent of the serotonin in your body. If your gut health is off, it can impact the production of serotonin, causing an imbalance of it in the brain, the hallmark of different mental health issues.

How's your gut health? Take the following assessment to find out.

To Test:

Read the following statements and answer yes or no to each.

1. **I experience frequent diarrhea (more than once a week).**
   Yes or No

2. I experience frequent constipation (less than one stool movement a day, more than once a week).
   Yes or No
3. My stomach frequently aches after I eat.
   Yes or No
4. I frequently feel bloated after a meal.
   Yes or No
5. I experience excessive belching.
   Yes or No
6. I experience excessive foul flatulence (gas).
   Yes or No
7. I suffer from frequent heartburn (sharp, burning, or like a tightening sensation in the chest, often a few hours after a meal).
   Yes or No
8. I feel groggy after eating.
   Yes or No
9. I have more than one food sensitivity (foods that upset my digestive system.)
   Yes or No

Scoring

If you answered yes to more than three statements, you may have gut issues that might need to be addressed by a health-care practitioner.

One thing you can try for yourself is an elimination diet. Start by removing all of the common food intolerances: dairy, gluten, corn, soy, eggs, and nuts. Also, eliminate any foods you think may be causing an issue for you in particular. See page 233 for how to follow an elimination diet.

STRESS

Stress is a necessary part of our lives and can have both beneficial and negative effects, depending on how we respond to an event, transition, or problem. The key to managing stress is to develop resilience. This term refers to the ability to *adapt* successfully in the face of stress, adversity, and other challenging circumstances, while maintaining physical and mental well-being.

You're resilient when you can handle the day-to-day trials and tribulations and bounce back after periods of deep struggle. We can't avoid challenging times; they're something we each experience throughout life. But, it's how we handle them that has the true impact on our well-being and quality of life. That's resilience.

This adaptive response is similar to the response your skin undergoes when you expose it to the sun. Imagine you have been living in a dark basement for three years. How much sun do you think it would take to stimulate skin adaptation and start getting a tan? Very little. How much sun does it take to burn you? Just a little bit more. This is why short, frequent exposure to the sun is the best way to tan if you are fair skinned. A single sunburn injures the skin and stops your progress.

When your body adapts—physically or mentally, it aims to become more resilient so that it doesn't suffer the same damage from the same activities or actions again. It is literally protecting itself from a potential insult in the future.

All stressors, regardless of where they come from—a hard workout, an argument with your spouse, or a job layoff—impact your ability to adapt to stress.

So, how do you build resilience to stress?

There are many ways—physical, mental, relational, and spiritual. Physically, exercise consistently, but without overdoing it. Eat a healthy, balanced diet to fortify yourself with nutrients that support physical and mental health. Make sure you get plenty of quality sleep. Cut down on alcohol and other drugs.

Mentally, realize that you're the only one who can control your fate. In other words, how you feel and the way you deal with a situation is a choice. Think of it like this: No one can operate your car unless you hand over the keys, right? You can't control other people's actions or behavior, but you can be responsible for how you react. Makes sense, right? Look at the situation and ask yourself, "Is this something I can change?" If so, start exploring positive ways to change the situation, or respond positively, and with acceptance, to the reality of your circumstances.

One of the biggest causations of stress has to do relationships. According to the American Institute of Stress, more than a quarter of people surveyed in 2014 felt alienated from a friend or family member because of stress, and over half had fought with people close to them.

This makes you wonder: How much of life stress is causing our relationship troubles? Research suggests that stress can indeed drive couples apart, but understanding how this happens may help them heal their relationships.

When you have healthy relationships, you have a support system that props you up when the going gets tough. You can share the stress of tough times as well as celebrate the joys of life with those around you.

Another aspect of life that can build resilience against stress is spirituality. It has many definitions, but generally it comes from your connection with others, your values, and your search for meaning in life. For many, spirituality involves religious worship, prayer, meditation, or a belief in a higher power. For others, it can be found in nature, music, or art. Spirituality is different for everyone.

Whatever the source, spirituality relieves stress by cultivating a sense of purpose in your life, connecting to people so that you feel less solitary, leading to greater inner peace, and releasing control. Studies have found that people who consider themselves spiritual may be better able to cope with stress and may experience health benefits.

What's your stress level? Let's take a short assessment to find out.

To Test:

Read the following statements and answer yes or no to each.

1. **I rarely get angry or tense because of things that are outside my control.**
   Yes or No

2. I rarely feel nervous and tense.
   Yes or No

3. I can cope with all the things I have to do.
   Yes or No

4. I rarely experience such symptoms as headaches, fatigue, tense muscles, difficulty falling asleep, or bouts of anger and hostility.
   Yes or No

5. I feel that I'm on top of things.
   Yes or No

6. I have a loving, satisfying relationship with my spouse or partner.
   Yes or No

7. I feel my life has purpose.
   Yes or No

8. I am connected to a spiritual community, or I have a strong social network.
   Yes or No

9. I create calmness in my life through the power of prayer or meditation.
   Yes or No

10. I have a daily practice of gratitude.
    Yes or No

11. I exercise at least three or four times a week.
    Yes or No

12. I do not abuse alcohol or drugs.
    Yes or No

13. If things aren't going well, I tend to view the situation as temporary rather than permanent.
    Yes or No

14. If I do get stressed, I can change my thinking to calm down.
    Yes or No

Scoring

If you answered no to five or more statements, you may have problems managing stress in your life. Engage in stress-reducing activities such as working out, meditating, prayer, going on long walks, and taking time away from work and obligations to relax. Recognize the source of your stress and take steps to mitigate it.

No matter what your scores were, feel encouraged! I've seen countless miracle transformations in people over the years as they continued on their paths to getting in shape. The same will happen to you as you start feeling, and looking, much better and healthier than you ever did before. The lifestyle changes you'll be making are sustainable and easily integrated into your current way of operating. This means that you'll be able to find time in your day for everything that is important to you and to mesh your fitness goals into that framework in a realistic, healthy, and balanced way.

4

SECRET WEAPONS TO
TRANSFORM YOUR BODY

L
ike many activities, resistance training has its own techniques,
even its own lingo. If you're new to resistance training, the
techniques and terms that get tossed around can be confusing
and overwhelming. Even though I've been at this a long time, I still
come across new terms and strategies that make me curious and want
to know more.

In this chapter, I cover terms and techniques that are not new. *But
what I have to say about them is new.* So, if you're past newbie status,
don't skip this chapter!

Resistance training must be done in a particular way. It's not just
a matter of hoisting weights around haphazardly. To gain the benefits that *only resistance training can provide*, you must pay attention to
the techniques you'll learn here. When you apply them, you create a
faster metabolism, stronger muscles, better mobility, and an increase
in lean muscle mass. All of this takes place when the body is properly
signaled to do so. It is an adaptation process. The techniques and
recommendations here are your secret weapons to make that happen.

REPETITIONS (REPS)

Every time you perform one movement sequence of an exercise, that
movement sequence is considered a repetition, or rep for short. If you

squat down and then go back up (a movement sequence), for example, you've performed one rep of a squat.

For developing muscle and strength, the ideal number of reps is between 5 and 30. Any more than 30 reps, and resistance training becomes more like cardio. This means you will get less of the desired muscle-building and metabolism-boosting benefits from your training. Very low reps have some value, however, but are best utilized by competitive lifters.

REPPING "TO FAILURE"—THIS COMMON MYTH WILL FAIL YOU!

There is a pervasive belief in the fitness world that you need to perform reps "to failure" to see significant progress. Reps to failure means you lift a weight or perform an exercise until you can no longer perform another good rep. You essentially go until you "fail."

Although lifting to failure may have some benefits for very advanced lifters when used sparingly, it should be completely avoided by the average person. Lifting to failure causes more damage than is needed to spur your body to change. With that level of damage, your body prioritizes recovery over adaptation.

Recovery is a healing process, whereas adaptation is the process by which your body becomes stronger and fitter. Training to failure is simply too much intensity for most people. It slows down progress and, in some cases, can actually put a halt to it.

When doing your reps, use an appropriate level of resistance for your individual body. If you are a beginner, you don't need to go very heavy at first to initiate changes. If you are intermediate to advanced, stop your reps at the point where you feel like you can maybe squeeze out two or three more reps before you "fail." This will result in faster and more consistent progress.

SETS

A *set* in resistance training is the term for the total number of consecutive repetitions (*reps*) you perform at one time. The number of sets and reps will vary according to (a) which workout plan you are following, (b) which exercise you are doing, and (c) how familiar you have become with that exercise.

We typically do multiple sets of an exercise rather than just one. Studies show that multiple sets of an exercise usually outperform single sets of an exercise. Throughout my years of training clients, I have found that three sets of an exercise is right around the sweet spot for most people. The first set gives your body an idea of what the movement is like and how you should perform it. The second set provides an opportunity to fine-tune the movement and apply a little more resistance. By the third set, you are ready to perform the exercise with your very best effort.

For example, following the chart on page 133, in the first phase of the Total Body Anywhere Workout, you will do one set of 5 to 20 reps of Bodyweight Squats in each workout session; in Phase 2, you will increase this to two sets of the same number of reps per set, and then in Phase 3, three sets of the same number of reps per set.

REST BETWEEN SETS

A certain amount of rest between sets is essential. Because resistance training emphasizes anaerobic ("without oxygen") metabolism, your muscles reach fatigue relatively quickly.

With resistance training, you primarily use fast-burning types of energy. One of these is known as adenosine triphosphate (ATP). This energy burns hot, but it also burns out rapidly. If you don't rest long enough to allow ATP to replenish, you will begin using slower types of energy. This results in more endurance than strength, essentially turning your resistance training workout into a cardio workout.

What's more, not resting in between sets may make your workouts feel harder, but it won't make them more effective. Resting in between sets is just as important as the sets themselves, so don't skip the rest period.

On average, I recommend one minute of rest between sets, sometimes longer based on your age or workout experience.

ROUTINE

A routine is the collection of resistance training exercises you perform each time you train. In other words, the "routine" is your workout. For the purposes of this book, you'll work your major muscle groups at a single session, or routine, two or three times a week.

Your workouts tell your body to adapt and change. The adaptation you're aiming for is fat loss, muscle and strength gains, and a faster metabolism. Of those three, the most important is a faster metabolism. If your metabolism is burning more calories at rest, this makes getting lean and staying lean much easier, especially since we live in a land of hyperplenty, calorie-dense processed foods. The routines in this book are designed to speed up your metabolism so that can create the body and health profile you want.

OVERLOAD

Overload is the amount of resistance, or weight, you use on sets. It is important to slightly increase overload from the previous set, or from the previous routine. Your muscles can then constantly adapt and become stronger.

Of course this adaptation must be appropriate to your current strength levels. Although it is desirable to be able to add a little more weight or reps each workout so as to "overload" your muscles, if you aren't yet strong enough to do so, then don't do it. At first, strength gains are linear, but over time, they happen at a slower pace and lessen in consistency. Just be patient and add weight or reps *when* appropriate.

Although muscles respond to any resistance, they *visibly* respond best to heavy resistance. For background, your muscles are made up of two general categories of muscle fibers: type 1 (slow-twitch) and type 2 (fast-twitch). Slow-twitch muscle fibers do well with cardio-style activity. When you are running for long periods of time, for instance, it's your slow-twitch muscle fibers that are affected the most. Fast-twitch muscle fibers, however, do well with heavy-type resistance work. It's the fast-twitch fibers that have the greatest capacity for growth and strength. This is why long-distance runners and cardio addicts have much less muscle in comparison to sprinters.

Heavy resistance, or overload, is individual. What is heavy for one person may be light for another. It simply needs to feel heavy for you to be effective.

RAW FITNESS TRUTH #4

TONED IS A MADE-UP WORD.

The fitness industry (like most industries) is driven by its marketing. The result of this has been decades of made-up words and false information designed to get people to buy exercise products, gym memberships, and supplements. Although both men and women are routinely lied to, the fitness industry takes special aim at the female market. This is likely due to the fact that women make up the majority of consumers in almost any market, and this is especially true in the fitness industry.

For example, I have a real problem with the word *toned*. I'm not sure who came up with this word, but I'm sure it was dreamed up to get women to buy gym memberships and workout videos. Muscles don't "tone." They either build or they shrink. As a muscle builds, it begins to feel harder—and it's this adaptation we typically refer to as "toning." Nonetheless, if your goal is to get a "toned" body, your goal should be to build muscle. In other words, the best "toning" workouts are the best muscle-building workouts.

I cringe when I look at the fitness programs directed at women. All of them promise to sculpt and "tone" without building huge muscles. The workouts typically use light weights or bands, short ranges of motion to promote a muscle burn, and very high reps. This approach is *terrible* for building muscle.

If you want to efficiently build muscle and improve your physique, your best bet is to lift heavier resistance and avoid the ineffective workouts and products that are marketed to women.

TEMPO

Tempo is the speed at which you perform each rep, including the lifting (concentric) phase and the lowering (eccentric) phase. The tempo I recommend is 2 to 4 seconds for the concentric phase, and 3 to 4 seconds for the eccentric phase. This pace allows for full control of the weight with no momentum.

Controlled tempo is ideal for strength and for muscle- and metabolism-boosting. It's also safer than fast or ballistic lifting. Going too slow (taking more than five seconds to go up or down) should also be avoided as well. When reps are done too slowly, they start to work more on endurance than on strength. Remember, you want strength because strength is what speeds up your metabolism.

TENSION

As you move through an exercise, it is important to keep tension on the working muscles for each and every set, and throughout the range of motion. This creates a very favorable environment for growth and tells your muscles to get stronger.

Continuous tension means that you keep your muscles flexed even when your joints are fully extended. An example would be at the top of a squat when you are standing up straight. Rather than resting at the top, you'd keep flexing the muscles to maintain tension.

MUSCLE CONTRACTIONS

Every resistance training exercise can be broken down into three main parts: the concentric phase, the eccentric phase, and the isometric phase of the movement. Focusing on each type can score you many benefits, from muscular development to flexibility.

Concentric. This phase happens when the muscle contracts, or shortens, and is typically the lifting portion of the exercise. The simplest example of a concentric movement is the biceps curl, in which you bring a dumbbell up from hip height to shoulder height. As the dumbbell gets closer to your shoulder, the biceps muscle shortens and the tension in the muscle increases. The concentric portion of a movement helps you build strength. (This movement is sometimes referred to as the "positive phase.")

Other common concentric movements include:

- Lifting an object off the ground
- Pressing to the top in a push-up
- Standing up during a squat
- The upward motion of a sit-up or a crunch

Eccentric. During the eccentric phase, you are lowering the resistance on each rep. Using the biceps curl example again, the eccentric movement happens while you lower the weight back down to hip level. This portion of the movement is just as important as the lifting movement because it triggers strength and muscle building. Eccentric training also strengthens your tendons and ligaments, thus decreasing your risk of injury. (This movement is sometimes referred to as the "negative phase.")

Other common eccentric movements include:

- Lowering yourself after pulling your chin above the bar in a pull-up
- Squatting down during a squat
- Slowly rolling back down during a crunch

Isometric. During an isometric move, you're literally holding completely still but with tension. There is no lengthening or shortening of the muscle. Not all exercises will include an isometric portion, but you can add one to most moves by pausing midway through the exercise.

Let's return to the biceps curl. You can apply isometric force by curling your biceps up to 90 degrees, so that your forearm is parallel to the floor, and then holding the dumbbell or barbell there for around five seconds. That's isometric training.

Like the other phases, isometrics force you to engage your muscles, make them stronger, and build lean muscle. Pausing also requires you to engage your core on most movements, so you can use isometrics to increase balance and body control.

Other common isometric movements include:

- Holding your body in a plank position
- Maintaining a chair pose in a yoga class
- Doing a wall sit, in which you move into a sitting position with your back against the wall and hold that position for as long as you can

INTENSITY

This term refers to how hard you work out and is typically based on the amount of resistance you use. No one disputes that a resistance training program must have a sufficient level of intensity to stimulate muscle growth. Unfortunately, intensity is also the most abused factor because people commonly assume that harder is better. Not true!

To be fair, intensity is important when you are trying to get your body to change. Intensity, however, feeds into the attitude of "all or nothing." You're probably familiar with this way of thinking, whether in your workouts or in other parts of your life. In short, it's the inclination to operate in extremes. Sometimes you're all-in, pushing hard at 110 percent through your exercises because you binged the night before, or you're calling it quits before you're even in your workout clothes. Extreme measures, either way, will not make you progress any faster and, in fact, may actually slow down your progress.

So, what is the right intensity?

My advice is this: When in doubt, for better and longer-lasting results, train at a low to moderate intensity rather than at a high intensity. In other words, there's no need to beat your muscles up, using superheavy resistance and training to failure. Also, when you use a low to moderate intensity, you can work out more often, if you can, and develop a superior physique.

Let me give you an example. Ever notice how muscular a mechanic's forearms are? Or the arms of a construction worker? How about the calves of a mail carrier or the upper body of a gymnast? These muscles were *not* simply built by superintense and infrequent workouts. Their muscles were largely built with lower intensity but more frequent use.

So, train at a low to moderate intensity, never go to failure, and do your workouts a few times a week—and you'll make amazing progress. The workouts in this book will help you apply the right intensity for the best results.

PRACTICE, DON'T WORK OUT

When you think of the words *work out*, what comes to mind? For most people, this term evokes images of sweating bodies, grunting and straining while lifting weights, or running or doing some other form of exercise with intensity. What if I told you that the most effective way to work out is not to place the focus on the "no pain, no gain" mantra (which is a myth) or the burn or how much sweat dripped off your body? What if I told you that true, effective working out is all about perfecting the skills instead of trying to make yourself sore?

Decades ago, when gyms first started popping up in America, they looked very different from the gyms we know and love today. There were no machines at all. They had rings, parallel bars, barbells, and dumbbells. Most of them didn't even have weight racks or benches. It was a far cry from the air-conditioned palaces we see today. They sure did look different, but the difference in appearance pales in comparison to the difference in how people approached exercise. I'm not talking about exercise selection or routines either (although that was also vastly different), I'm referring to the entire approach to the concept of exercise.

SORENESS IS A TERRIBLE INDICATOR OF A GOOD WORKOUT.

To be honest, there is a lot of debate as to what exactly causes muscle soreness. We know there is some inflammation and some muscle damage, but otherwise, we really aren't too sure. Any exercise or routine outside of your normal training can cause soreness. I train my body with weights on a very regular basis and at an advanced level, but if I were to go swim for a mile, I can assure you I would be sore the next day.

Does this mean that the swim stimulated more strength and muscle growth than my regular weight training workouts? No, not all. Soreness does not mean you stimulated progress toward greater muscle development. If you are sore to the touch, or the soreness lasts longer than one or two days, it is likely that you overapplied intensity and trained way too hard. Applying too much intensity will not get you to your goals faster; it will get you there much more slowly.

On the other hand, you might be a little sore after a workout. That is okay. Just be aware that long-lasting excessive soreness is not a good thing.

The only way to tell whether a workout is effective is your progress, plain and simple. Are you getting stronger? Are your muscles more defined? Do you have less body fat? If the answers are yes to all questions, then congratulations, you are training effectively. If your answers are no, then I am sorry to tell you that what you are doing is not working, regardless of how sore you get.

What should you do if you get sore after a workout? Answer: light movement. Above all, do not lie around and become sedentary, thinking you need to nurse your sore muscles, or else you will start to lose that muscle. You can resume your workouts, but train with less intensity—with lighter resistance and greater frequency, for example. Low-intensity exercise actually speeds up and facilitates recovery.

People did not go to these gyms to sweat, get a pump, feel their muscles burn, get sore, or burn calories. Instead, patrons went to learn skills and to practice these skills. It was very similar to learning how to play a new sport. If you wanted to learn how to play baseball, you wouldn't just get on a field and swing like mad trying to burn calories and get sore, you would practice and learn the skills necessary to play the game properly.

Then, the attitude started to shift around exercise. The skill of exercise became an afterthought and the side effect of looking fit became the main focus. It wasn't about learning how to squat perfectly; it became about getting the legs sore. It wasn't about perfecting lifts anymore; it became about looking like you could lift. Although I completely understand the preoccupation with looks (heck, that is the main reason that I started working out), it's the unintended consequences of this attitude that have made working out less effective and much less safe.

Here is a good example of what I am talking about. Thousands of Americans take up running every single year in their pursuit of fat loss. Most of them are almost complete beginners, and the rest of them haven't run consistently for years. They just pick up and decide, "That's it, I need to get in shape," and then go outside and start running. The goal is not to run well at all, the goal is to sweat and burn calories.

Running is a very complex skill that requires daily practice to perform properly. When people haven't run for years, and they decide it's time to run, it takes months or years of proper running practice, correctional exercises, and stretching to get them to be able to run efficiently. If these people get out and start running with the intent of just sweating, then form and technique no longer matter. Even worse, they run to fatigue (because they just want a "workout") and when a body fatigues, form gets even worse. This is why running causes thousands of injuries a year. It's not because running is dangerous (we evolved to run); rather, it is because bad running is dangerous.

It would be much more effective for these people to practice running instead of running to work out. They would still burn calories, but they would also greatly reduce risk of injury. Over time, they would slowly perfect how they ran to the point where they could simply run for a "workout."

The same is true for resistance training. I've never heard a gym member say, "I want to learn how to squat properly." Instead, it was "I want to get a good workout to get fit." This is a huge mistake. Starting off with that mentality means people value soreness, sweat, and perceived effort above all else. It means that form really is just an afterthought. If only these people understood that practicing exercise would get them far better and longer-lasting results.

Next time you start your workout, especially if you're new to resistance training, start it with a mentality to practice exercise. Look at every movement in your workout the same way athletes look at their sports. It's a skill. Practice and perfect the movements and go hard, but never so hard that your form breaks down and you lose skill. You will find that workouts are more enjoyable, you don't beat your body up so much, and your body will progress more consistently. Well-executed and connected movement produces better results than poorly executed and disconnected movements even if the intensity is lower. Practice, don't work out.

THE BEST GYM IS A HOME GYM

The resistance training workouts in this book are designed to be performed at home. Home gyms have some major advantages over commercial gyms. The biggest is convenience. Having to drive to a commercial gym, park, change in the locker room and then drive home afterward can add fifteen minutes or more to your schedule. With a home gym, you just work out. Zero travel time.

If you have kids at home, you can just put them down for a nap or in a play pack and do your workout. One reason I love working out at home is that my children watch me, and this sets a good example. You can even exercise with a partner, such as your spouse or your teenager. This gets everyone into the act.

Another advantage is in the comfort. At a commercial gym, you are around other people. This means you can't work out shirtless, barefoot, or in old hole-filled sweats. At home, you can wear whatever you want. And you don't have to feel self-conscious around people who are lifting huge amounts of weight to show off.

At home, you can also blast whatever music you want. Music is motivating and has a significant effect on how well you work out. In a study published in 2010, researchers found that when people listened to faster music, it motivated them to increase the intensity of their workouts. Music can really fire up your workouts.

You can also yell while deadlifting, perspire all over your own equipment and not have to worry about other people's sweat and germs, and you can walk right into your kitchen after you lift to eat a postworkout meal.

You might think that one disadvantage of home training is the lack of the huge variety of equipment. But guess what? That really isn't a disadvantage unless you get bored without tons of variety.

Not only is most of this fancy gym equipment unnecessary, but it also won't give you any better results than if you stuck with the most basic free weight equipment: that is, barbells or dumbbells that are not attached to a machine.

Why do gyms buy all that stuff? Because it doesn't look cool if the resistance training area consisted of only barbells, dumbbells, benches, and squat racks. They wouldn't sell as many memberships.

The top five best exercises for every body part are either entirely free weight exercises or mostly free weight exercises. These exercises include barbell squats, deadlifts, bench presses, overhead presses, rows, walking lunges, barbell curls, and triceps extensions—all of which you'll learn to do in this book. Due to their muscle- and strength-building power, they are also amazing metabolism boosters and fat burners.

So, all in all, home gyms are the best, and in my experience, people who work out at home are much more consistent.

HOW TO SET UP YOUR HOME GYM

Since I started doing resistance training at age fourteen, I have mostly worked out at home, despite managing gyms and training people. My dad bought a decent home gym setup back then. In our backyard, under the patio cover, he set up a sturdy bench that adjusted to an incline, a barbell, two adjustable dumbbells, a curl bar, and more than 300 pounds of Olympic free weights. It was a pretty cool setup at the time. I lifted weights entirely in that backyard with that equipment for a little over two years and made some amazing progress.

When I owned my personal training studio, I had just a bit more than that original backyard iron set, namely a full squat rack and some cables. I ultimately developed the best physique of my life using only that equipment.

I still primarily use very basic equipment and do 80 percent of my workouts in my small garage. I have a gym membership, but I prefer to work out at home most of the time.

Here is all you need to set up a great home gym, do the workouts in this book, and be able to train your entire body effectively and at any level of training:

Barbells and dumbbells (free weights). A barbell is a steel bar measuring 4 to 6 feet in length. Some barbells have a fixed amount of weight on the sides; other barbells allow you to add and subtract weight (a.k.a. plates) as you wish.

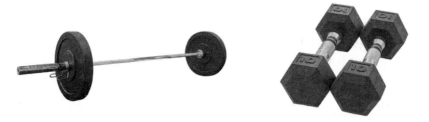

Made of steel or heavy rubber, dumbbells are smaller versions of barbells that can be used individually or in pairs, with one in each hand. It's a good idea to purchase a set of dumbbells of varying poundages so that you can progressively increase your resistance when working out.

Free weights allow your body to lift and move in natural ways, whereas machines dictate the way the body must move. Free weights thus provide a stability component that translates into better results. Plus, there are hundreds of exercises that you can do with free weights.

In the real world, you're lifting things that are free, such as boxes or furniture. Using free weights strengthens your body for real-life daily activity.

A squat rack. This is a steel apparatus that lets you do weighted squats safely, as well as other forms of exercises, such as bench presses.

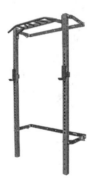

An adjustable bench. A bench provides a designated spot to use your weights or practice many different exercises. Make sure to get one that can transition from a flat position to an inclined position. Exercises performed on an incline or decline put different stresses on muscles for greater progress.

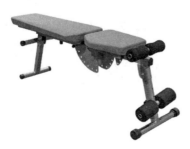

A calf block. This is a small raised platform on which you can do calf raises to develop, stretch, and shape your calf muscles. Alternatively, you can use a stair on your staircase. This works just as well.

A stability ball. This tool is a soft, lightweight ball that ranges in diameter and is designed to stretch and develop the abs, which are part of the body's core. (More on stability balls on page 111.)

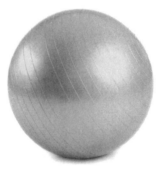

A sturdy box. This piece of equipment is simply a stable box or platform on which you can perform "step-ups." This exercise involves stepping up and down onto a box or platform. It works the thighs and glutes. Make sure you find a box that won't move out from under you when you step up onto it.

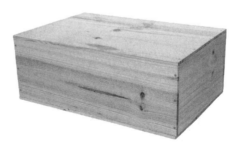

Resistance bands. These are available in a variety of resistance levels: light, medium, and heavy. It's a good idea to purchase all three levels to be able to make progress and work out with the appropriate intensity. If you are new to resistance training, it is a good idea to start with bands. (More on resistance bands on page 110.)

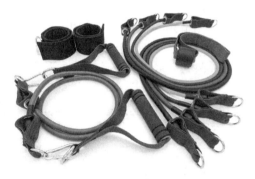

An exercise mat. Purchase a lightweight mat that rolls up easily. Mats help cushion your knees and back while doing floor exercises.

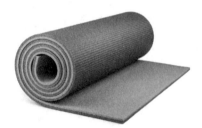

Your own bodyweight. Bodyweight exercises use your own weight to provide resistance. Otherwise known as "equipment-free" training, bodyweight workouts can give you an effective fat-burning and muscle-building workout when you don't have access to free weights.

I never totally believed this until I met a personal trainer named Zach, who once used my personal training facility to train his clients. Zach had some seriously muscular and advanced male and female clients. Although the high fitness level of his clients was out of the ordinary (most personal training clients are average people), I was mostly intrigued by how he trained his clients. He almost never used any weights or equipment whatsoever.

I was perplexed so I asked him about his training methodology and practices. "Why don't you ever use any equipment with your clients?"

He responded, "I was a competitive gymnast for years, and I understand the value of bodyweight movements for function and for muscular development. It works great for me and for my clients."

Zach was exactly right. Take a look at high-level gymnasts. They have some of the most muscular and balanced physiques on the planet. The amount of balance and control it takes to perform many bodyweight movements engages support muscles and stabilizers like crazy. Over time, your whole body can develop in ways that reflect your ability to control and lift your own body—simply by using bodyweight exercises.

Bodyweight routines are excellent for beginners, but they also benefit people with workout experience. You can even increase your intensity when doing bodyweight workouts. For example, doing a push-up is hard enough by itself, but if you wanted to make it even harder and more challenging, try doing a one-arm push-up! Or you can make bodyweight exercises more intense by increasing your reps.

One of the workouts in Part 2 is a serious bodyweight routine with fat-burning and muscle-building benefits. It is appropriate for beginners and for anyone with at least one year of workout experience under their belt. Zach made a believer out of me, and I hope this workout will do the same for you.

Finally, if you want to get really fancy, purchase a basic cable setup for triceps pressdowns or lat pulldowns. But even without it, you have access to hundreds of free weight exercises, and you can effectively train your entire body. If you are serious about fitness and want to see amazing gains with intense workouts and also value privacy and convenience, a home gym is the way to go. You won't be disappointed.

Before we move into the actual resistance training exercises, routines, and nutrition plan, I want to make sure you develop the right mindset. Yes, you've got to condition your body, but you've got to condition your mind first. That's where we're headed next.

5

DO YOU REALLY WANT IT?

What gets you to exercise, eat right, or switch to a healthier lifestyle, let alone stick with it?

How do you get started to be able to experience the joy of being fit and strong?

What does it take to stay engaged for the year ahead—and indeed, for a lifetime?

Do you really want to stay in top-notch shape and enjoy great health for as long as you can?

Working in gyms and training clients for a long time, I was always puzzled about these questions—and the answers. I witnessed person after person come into my gyms with amazing enthusiasm, buy memberships, hire trainers, and start with gusto, only to completely disappear a few months later.

What gives? I'd ask myself. Fully dedicated to helping people succeed, I made it my mission to figure all this out.

First, I wanted to understand why such seemingly motivated people could just quit their fitness and health journeys. Second, and most important, I wanted to know why other people did *not* quit and how they developed long-term fitness and health habits.

After years of observing, questioning, and working intently with people, I now have answers. Some of them might surprise you, so strap in for a wild ride.

MOTIVATION VERSUS DISCIPLINE

A lot of people say, "I need to get motivated," or "I just don't have the motivation." Understand right away that motivation is a *feeling*. Like any feeling, it is not permanent. Motivation is short term, and usually fleeting. It waxes and wanes.

When we feel motivated, we tend to overestimate our abilities and feel that we can do anything. If we *always* felt that motivated, getting in shape would be easy. You eat right or work out consistently when you feel temporarily charged up. But like a fair-weather friend, motivation isn't always there for you when you need it. As soon as motivation fades, which it inevitably will, your new lifestyle is impossible to maintain.

So, what can keep you moving toward your goals, living a fit lifestyle, even on days when you don't feel like it—when you're not motivated?

Answer: Discipline with a capital D!

When it comes to sustaining a lifetime of strength and fitness, it's a rock-solid discipline that will carry you to new heights—and keep you there.

But what's the difference between motivation and discipline? Maybe you thought they were one and the same. Not at all. Remember, motivation is a *feeling*. It occurs in bursts. But discipline is a *skill*—an acquired ability that is self-perpetuating and constant. Big difference.

The key is to not rely on motivation but to rely on discipline. It is the catalyst to sustained action and ongoing energy for motion—it propels you to *stick to something as a matter of habit and follow through*. The perfect plan for lifelong fitness is of no use in the absence of discipline.

Here's the best part: like all skills, you can develop discipline, and it's not that hard.

All you have to do is give yourself one challenging but realistic goal that is failproof. Rather than say, "I will go to the gym five days a week"—which is unrealistic, set a goal to go one or two days a week.

I've had clients who could realistically commit to only thirty minutes a week, so we'd work with that half hour. They would start feeling good after the workout. Eventually, they'd be ready for a full hour each week. Then another and another, until they were getting more physical activity under their belt. And while this was getting them back into shape, it was also building a daily habit that helped them graduate to more intense programs in the future.

So, you see: Little by little, they developed the skill of discipline, and they did not want to stop working out. In fact, those clients who developed discipline and relied on it over motivation, every single one of them is still working out faithfully six to twelve years after we started.

Discipline works equally well when it comes to nutrition. I once had a client who was the most unhealthy person ever. She never drank any water, only diet cola. I suggested that we come up with a simple, attainable goal: drink one glass of water a day. That's where we started.

She drank a glass of water each day until it became easy. Then, we added another glass and another glass. Once she acquired the discipline of drinking more water, we moved on to another goal: eliminating one can of soda a day until that became easy. Then, we gradually cut out more cans of soda. When she was ready, we did the same thing with vegetables. She'd eat one serving of vegetables a day until she was ready to add more.

By the end of one year, she had lost 20 pounds and was working out twice a week. She looked amazing, but more than that, she fell in love with feeling healthy and fit. She did not want to give that up. By developing the skill of discipline, she became a lifelong health and fitness convert.

A lot of people want to get lean and fit fast. That's all they care about. But it can't all happen at once.

Permanent change comes slowly. If someone painted two parallel lines on a highway but moved one of the lines up a tiny degree farther from parallel with each stroke, the distance between the lines would be barely noticeable. But 2 miles down the road, you'd see how far apart they are. That's the nature of lasting change. It comes slowly but is permanent.

Maintaining discipline is about keeping your mind on the prize. Know what you're working toward and stick to your plan for getting there. Take things one day at a time, and one step at a time. This gives you little victories that boost your confidence and collectively develop discipline that will last you a lifetime.

SMALL GOALS, BIG WINS

Allow me to elaborate on goal setting a bit, and give you my take. When you do feel that surge of motivation, you decide, once and for all, "It's time to do something about this!"

That surge propels you to set huge, out-of-reach goals for yourself. It was not uncommon for new gym members to tell me their fitness goals were to lose 30-plus pounds, and the time frame was usually "as fast as possible." They meant it too. They were ready to work out five days a week, hire me, buy a boatload of supplements, and completely revamp their diet. If this sounds like you, don't feel bad. You aren't alone. This describes most of us at one time or another.

Setting goals in a very motivated mind-set is not a good idea. It is destined to fail for the reasons I explained earlier.

It's better to be completely honest and ask yourself the following question: "What can I start now that I know I can and will maintain forever?" Answer this question with brutal honestly and make sure to use *forever* as your context. Pick a small goal that is challenging (this gives it meaning) but also honestly realistic.

What you will find is that your goals and the methods you decide to employ to accomplish those goals change immediately. This is not only perfectly fine, but it's also awesome because you now have attainable goals. No goal is too small here, and there is no such thing as too little exercise or too few dietary changes as long as they are more than you are doing now.

If you aren't exercising at all now, for example, then even one day a week is an improvement. If you pay zero attention to your diet, then simply being more conscious of your junk food intake is an excellent place to start.

Now you have a great starting point with your goals, but we aren't done. Deep down inside, you really do want to lose a lot of body fat. You really do want to live a healthy, vibrant life. You achieve these benefits from a lifelong healthy relationship with exercise and nutrition.

So, what do we do after we become consistent with our initial small goals and realistic methods? Repeat the process! Once your new realistic goal has been achieved and has solidified as a behavior of yours, have the honest conversation with yourself again. Make another small, challenging, but realistic goal, rinse and repeat!

These small but permanent changes equate to *huge* changes over time. I have seen dramatic transformations with this method, and the best part is that most of them were permanent.

RAW FITNESS TRUTH #6

YOU *DO* HAVE TIME TO WORK OUT.

The most common excuse I've heard for not working out is: "I don't have time." Nine out of ten times, people blame lack of time. We're all busy, sometimes, too busy to get in some moderate exercise our body needs daily to stay fit.

Whenever someone told me they didn't have time, I would go into my motivational spiel in which I'd ask them to list their life priorities on a piece of paper. Inevitably, they'd acknowledge that health was their number one concern. After all, without good health, you can't work, take care of your kids, or live life in the ways you truly want to.

continues

continued

Back then, my solution to the "time" excuse was to motivate and inspire people to instantly prioritize their health by taking hours out of their week to drive to my gym and work out.

This approach worked great—in the short term. Most people did get motivated and inspired, and they did get results—at first. The problem was that eventually they stopped their consistent workouts and became a part of the statistic that shows that most people who start a fitness program eventually stop.

I had to be honest with myself: I wasn't really helping anyone. It was at this point that I realized I had to meet people where they are.

Many people do have crazy schedules, and they are slammed with responsibilities. When you factor in family time, work, household duties, and more, it can be very daunting to go from not going to the gym to dedicating four to five hours a week to exercise (time it takes driving to and from, plus time in the gym working out).

I needed to come up with a solution. I had to design workouts that were extremely convenient. They needed to be effective with minimal time. So, that's what I did.

I went on to create workouts that took a grand total of 90 minutes per week. These workouts were targeted at two types of busy people: the type who wants to work out only a few days a week and the other who wants to work out a little bit most days. They had the option of doing three 30-minute workouts or six 15-minute workouts a week. This total time even included mobility work to prevent injury and to encourage better body mechanics.

As it turned out, the workouts did their job (with diet). They increased muscle mass, burned fat, and increased metabolism. They were also very effective at building consistency, which led to helping clients eventually progress to spending more time working out and maybe even joining a gym. And of course, they proved to be very successful in helping stay-at-home parents,

continues

continued

business travelers, and other busy people get in shape over the short and long term.

The truth is you can get great fitness results with as little as a grand total of 60 minutes a week of dedicated workout time. In fact, that amount of exercise may even add years to your life. According to a study in the journal *Medicine and Science in Sports and Exercise*, burning only 1,000 calories a week through exercise reduced the risk of dying prematurely. The study emphasized that some activity is better than none, but more is also better than some.

The key is also to make the workout as effective as possible— not "as hard as possible." The workouts you're about to learn are based on these principles: they're time efficient, they get results, and they can be done in the convenience of your home.

"I CAN'T" VERSUS "I DON'T WANT"

"I can't eat that" or "I have to work out." These are very common phrases people say when they are trying to get in shape or improve their fitness, and I've heard them all the time. I've even uttered them myself, especially after someone would ask me whether I wanted to indulge in a food that I knew was counter to my fitness goals. That was before I smartened up a bit as a personal trainer.

The first half of my career I learned all about proteins, fats, and carbs. I understood all about calories in versus calories out. I could re-cite information on biomechanics and exercise technique. I obsessed about these things and became somewhat of an expert. Yet had I been truly honest with myself, I wasn't really helping a majority of my clients.

Many clients back then would see some success with me and then would waver, plateau, and stay stuck. If any of them stopped training with me, then it was just a matter of time before they got right back to where they were before they met me. It was incredibly frustrating for me because I really wanted to see my clients achieve permanent, long-lasting success.

The second half of my career, this situation got under my skin so badly that I became entirely frustrated with fitness. Why couldn't I help these people? Were they just lazy? This is when I decided to dig much deeper.

I started to focus on the "why" instead of the "how." I already knew how people could get themselves in shape. In other words, I knew the process and the steps, but what eluded me was why they just didn't follow them. What could I do as a trainer to get people to make long-lasting changes? What were the "blocks" that stopped people from achieving goals they sincerely wanted to achieve? One day while at a family function, it came to me.

"Hey, Sal, have a piece of cake," my cousin yelled at me from across the room. My family knew I ate a very regimented diet, but they always tried to convince me to go off the rails. "No thanks, man. You know I can't eat that" was my reply. Then, he came back with the typical "Oh, come on man, it's just one piece; you will still be fit and lean tomorrow." He kept persisting, until I finally told my cousin, "I don't want the cake."

This response worked like magic, and he left me alone. "That's interesting," I thought. When I said that I couldn't *have* the cake, it was a debate. But when I said I didn't *want* the cake, he left me alone.

Why did changing my phrase work so well? Then the more important question came to me . . . why do I always say I can't eat something? Of course, I can eat something . . . unless someone is forcing me. "Wait a minute," I thought, "I am forcing myself." Boom, everything became clear.

Whenever we decide something is important, we make a plan to follow through. If the plan is especially challenging, we literally create two identities within ourselves. The first identity is the person who needs to lose weight or get in shape and so forth. The other identify is the dictator who *forces* us to follow through with the plan.

The dictator can be quite effective in the short term as long as we force ourselves to do things we feel we don't want to do, but disastrous in the long term because no one wants to be oppressed for the rest of their lives.

Think about it: how many times have you done this to yourself? One of you forces the other to obey. This works until the side of you that you identify with finally can't take any more oppression, and you rebel. You're strict until you decide "screw this" and you "go off the rails" or "fall off the wagon," and it's usually in a very big way. It's not just one small bite of cake, it's two whole pieces. It's not one or two missed workouts, it's quitting for months or years.

This behavior is largely due to perception. Perceive it as tyranny, and you will eventually rebel. Perceive it as something you choose to do and want to do, and there is nothing to rebel against.

Personally, I never had an issue with diet and exercise, but I did have a major problem with household chores. I hated them. I was raised in a very old-school stereotypical Sicilian family in which my mom did everything in the house. I rarely made a bed or washed a dish growing up. In fact, the few times I did do things around the house, it was because I was being punished. So, as an adult, I identified doing house chores as a punishment (similar to how people view eating healthy and exercising). I couldn't stand doing them, and, as a result, I contributed very little in this regard.

Once I realized that I wasn't being forced; rather, I actually wanted to do these things (I liked a clean, organized house), I changed how I perceived things. I realized that I only felt forced because there was a second version of myself—the dictator—who would tyrannize me to do things around the house. With that realization, I eliminated that version of myself who lived in my mind and simply realized that I wanted to do these things. Instantly they became less arduous and, in fact, became meditative at times.

I started teaching this concept to my clients, and their results dramatically improved. The best part was that they started experiencing far less stress and anguish over working out and eating right. Once they realized that they actually wanted to exercise and eat right, the rest was easy.

Do away with that other tyrannical version of yourself. Stop forcing yourself with "I can'ts." When you say no to a particular food, it is because you don't want it. Sure, you like how it tastes, and you might enjoy it momentarily, but you don't want to trade that for how it will make you feel or how it will impact your health. When you work out it's not because you have to; rather, it's because you want to. Sure, it will hurt a bit and is challenging, but it's worth all the benefits you want to happen to your body and health.

The same is true when you decide you do want to skip a workout day or if you actually do want to eat that piece of cake (or other food). On those occasions, you will realize that it's not that you are "going off the wagon" or that "you are rebelling"; rather, you don't mind the trade-off at that moment and you truly want to. This simple understanding reframes what actually drives you to make fitness and health decisions and eliminates the stress, failure, and self-blame that accompanies them.

SELF-LOVE VERSUS SELF-HATE

I always wanted my clients to succeed, while always trying to understand why some lapsed. Yes, it had to do with the issues I have just discussed, but it also had to do with how they felt about themselves.

Many of those who lapsed lacked a loving attitude toward their body. If "haters" binged on a dinner of nachos and burritos, for example, they'd head to the gym the next day and pummel themselves with exercises as a form of punishment. That's the dictator coming out again.

When you train yourself like this—out of self-hate—it is not effective. Nor will it sustain a lifetime of health and fitness.

Although hating your body is a powerful motivator initially, it will eventually drive you to make decisions that aren't in your best interest. Here is another example: Imagine you hate your belly. To you, it's disgusting, ugly, and you just want it gone. You are angry with yourself for even letting yourself get a belly.

So, you force yourself to go to the gym. You perform some kind of insane, intense workout because you hate your belly. In essence, you're punishing yourself out of hate.

The attitude of hating eventually demotivates you. At some point, you get sick of hating your body. Next, your motivation fades because it's just a feeling, and you just want to feel good. You fall off the wagon and say, "Screw it, I just want to love myself now and feel good." So, you stop all exercise and you binge on your favorite foods. *Does this cycle sound familiar?* You simply cannot make the best decisions if you hate yourself.

In fact, many people who hate themselves and their body decide to follow self-destructive paths to look good. They go on extreme diets. They take anabolic steroids to build muscle. They undergo one plastic surgery procedure after another. They might look temporarily good, but over time, these choices can ultimately lead to poor health and poor looks.

Put another way, good health looks good. Bad health looks bad. Pursue health through self-love and the looks will follow. Pursue looks through self-hate and your health will eventually suffer and you will lose the looks.

So, train yourself out of self-love. Practice saying: "How can I take care of myself in the gym with exercise?" Repeat this over and over in your mind, and it will move you from self-hate to self-love—and ultimately a healthier, more amazing-looking body and a powerfully positive mental health.

Once I started teaching my clients to train and eat because they love their body instead of hate it, their results were amazing. Clients succeeded faster, and their success seemed more effortless. They also stayed fit and healthy. Their techniques and training methods didn't change, but how they applied them did.

Let's use a different example. Say you look in the mirror, and you objectively notice that you haven't been taking good care of the only body you have. This does not make you a bad or disgusting person. In fact, at this moment, you realize how much you *love* yourself and want to start taking care of yourself.

Now, when you go to the gym, you work out because you *love* your body. You eat healthy foods because you *love* your body. You follow a healthy lifestyle routine with good sleep and stress management because you *love* your body.

Also, "love" does not necessarily mean "like." Sometimes, I don't like my kids, but I always love them. Loving your body simply means you want to take *care* of your body. It also allows you to separate self-image from body image. It is okay to look in the mirror and notice you have excess body fat or that you need more strength, but that does not mean you are a bad person or that you don't deserve respect.

Ask yourself this question: *If I truly enjoy working out and eating right, can I sustain these behaviors for a lifetime?* Of course, you can. Once you make this shift in how you think about exercise and diet, the rest is easy. Switching your focus to loving yourself will give you the breakthrough you need. You'll discover that healthy looks good on you.

APPEARANCE VERSUS HEALTH

Of all of the reasons people give for beginning or maintaining a fitness regime, the most popular by far is to improve the appearance of their body. I would even venture to say that if exercise did nothing to improve appearance but still provided all of the other benefits, such as improving health, increasing mobility, reducing stress, building strength, and so forth, gyms and fitness classes would lose 70 to 80 percent of their members. This isn't necessarily a bad thing, but it does provide us with valuable information that can help all of us with how we value fitness and how much we prioritize it in our everyday lives.

I am also confident that the remaining minority—20 to 30 percent of the people who currently work out—would stay with it, regardless.

The secret to long-term success with fitness lies within that minority group.

The secret, of course, is consistency. Even a subpar workout program done consistently is far more effective than the best and well-planned workout that is done inconsistently.

There are many factors that can contribute to consistency, but chief among them is the core reason you work out. Focusing on appearance as the main driver will prevent you from developing a good relationship between you and exercise and, often times, will result in *worse* results even if you still work out consistently. The best long-term approach is to value exercise for all its other benefits. This will lead to consistency, which will then lead to better aesthetic results. Ironically, not focusing on appearance will give you better chances at improving your appearance through fitness.

Keep the following in mind: a healthy body looks good; an unhealthy body does not. Make looks the primary focus and oftentimes you will sacrifice your health (through unhealthy dieting, overtraining, "punishment" dieting, exercising, etc.) for the pursuit of appearance; as your health declines, so will your appearance. Make health your primary focus and the looks will follow.

More so than any other factor, more than knowledge—even more than the perfect plan—discipline, realistic goal setting, and mind-set determine your success in fitness and in life. Do you really want those things? If so, tap into the power of these abilities and step into your best, healthiest future.

PART 2

WORKOUTS THAT MAXIMIZE METABOLISM, HEALTH, AND LONGEVITY

6

THE POWER OF PRIMING— GET RESISTANCE-READY!

With the workouts and guidelines in this part of the book, the number one goal is adaptation, so that you keep making progress without plateaus. Adaptation means continual muscle development, strength, fat loss, greater mobility, athleticism, and ultimately better health and improved aesthetics. Without the proper muscular adaptation signals, your body will actually avoid developing muscle and losing weight. Thus, each workout makes adaptation the sole focus of the programs.

ADAPTATION STARTS WITH PROPER "PRIMING"

Priming is the first component of all the *Resistance Training Revolution* workouts. This refers to specialized exercises designed to activate the adaptation process. *There is a difference between priming and warming up.*

When I became a personal trainer, my first certification courses paid little attention to warm-ups. We were told that a warm muscle was more "pliable;" therefore, it was best to get the muscles "warm" with some cardio and to do some long-hold stretches ("static stretching") prior to moving into a workout. And so, this approach is what the vast majority of we trainers did with our clients.

Then some scientific data surfaced that turned everything on its ear. Studies were published showing that static stretching prior to a workout actually *increased* the rate of injury and also reduced power output and athletic performance. This new information ran 180 degrees counter to what we all thought was common knowledge.

We learned that static stretching sends a signal to your central nervous system that says, "Relax this muscle and send a weaker signal to it." This is fine if you are going to lie down or relax after static stretching, but it is not a good thing if you want to work out and activate your muscles. A "relaxed" muscle from a static stretch has less strength and stability, and this increases risk of injury.

So, the conventional practice of warming up is not at all what it's cracked up to be. Fortunately, we now have a better option: priming. Not only does proper priming reduce injury risk, but it also increases functional ranges of motion, improves immediate strength output, improves overall performance, and makes your workouts more effective. Priming your body tells your central nervous system to fire muscles in ways that are beneficial for your individual body—and sets up your muscles for your workout.

Here is an example. Let's say I have a client who has poor posture in the form of forward-sloping shoulders. This situation looks just like it sounds: shoulders rounded forward. It's a very common posture issue these days, especially in people who spend hours each day slumped over their computer and at a desk.

If I took this client through a squat or a bench press, that posture would compromise his or her positioning, power, and the overall effectiveness of the workout. Take the barbell squat, for instance. An effective and efficient barbell squat has many moving parts, and all of them influence one another. To execute the squat properly, you have to maintain a tall posture with shoulder blades squeezed back and down, and your hands placed firmly on the bar. If any of these points are compromised by poor posture, your upper back tends to roll forward, and strength output is reduced. Less weight can be lifted, and less muscle is built. A forward posture also increases the risk of lower back rounding, which increases the risk of injury.

In this example, my client can "prime" by performing some light band rows, in which the focus is on squeezing the shoulders back and down. This signals the central nervous system to get into the best position for barbell squats. Priming thus results in better results and performance because ideal movement is achieved in a shorter period of time. Priming makes your workout safer and more effective—both of which support continued muscle development.

So, when you follow one of the workouts in this book, you can expect faster results with less work. More muscle, more rapid fat loss, and ongoing, perpetual progress . . . that's the *Resistance Training Revolution* way.

You'll be introduced to four workouts in this part of the book:

The Total Body Anywhere Program. I designed this program specifically for the beginner who has little to no experience with resistance training or who hasn't trained consistently for a few years. It is geared toward increasing strength, developing muscle, and improving overall health, stability, and mobility and comes with a full workout breakdown that tells you exactly what to do for your workouts throughout an entire nine-week period. All you need are resistance bands, a stability ball, and your own bodyweight. If you are a beginner, start here. Best of all, you can do this workout anywhere.

This chapter also includes the Mobility Program. As a reminder, mobility is foundational to success, and everyone should do mobility training. This program provides exercises you can work into any of the workouts, depending on your physical needs.

The Total Body Dumbbell Program. Here, all you'll need are dumbbells in different poundages or adjustable to different weights, and an adjustable exercise bench. This workout is also appropriate for beginners, as well as intermediate exercisers. It is also perfect to do at home or on the go. So, pick up those dumbbells and get to work!

The Total Body Home Gym Program. If your current fitness level is intermediate or advanced, and you have set up a home gym, this is the workout for you. You'll want to have barbells, dumbbells, an adjustable exercise bench, and a squat rack in your home gym for this program.

All of these programs are designed to systematically build strength, fitness, and aesthetics. *Select one program* and follow it consistently, as described, before moving on to another one. Jumping out of a program into another one that looks more "sexy" is like pulling a pie out of the oven before it's done. So, stay with your chosen program the full nine weeks!

LEVEL OF RESISTANCE TRAINING EXPERIENCE

You will always get the best results if you follow a routine that is appropriate for your individual body. Doing too much will result in *worse* progress. You can't fast-forward your strength gains, muscle development, and fat loss by jumping into a program that is too advanced for your current level.

So, before you start, figure out what your weight training experience level is. Is yours:

- *Beginner:* 0–2 months of consistent weekly resistance training experience
- *Intermediate:* 3–6 months of consistent weekly resistance training experience
- *Advanced:* over 6 months of consistent weekly resistance training experience

The reason you must identify this beforehand is that there are many differences among the three workouts in terms of what you're capable of doing and what will work best for you.

RESISTANCE TRAINING GUIDELINES

1. The programs are divided into Workout 1 and Workout 2. Ideally, they should be done every week with two days of rest in between. For example, you could do Workout 1 on Monday and Workout 2 on Thursday. You also have the option to do three workouts a week. In that case, alternate between Workout 1 and Workout 2, with one day of rest in between. A good workout schedule would be Monday, Wednesday, and Friday.

2. Begin each workout with "primers"—targeted and effective "priming movements." In the exercise descriptions, I provide detailed instructions for various types of priming movements.

3. Each program lasts nine weeks. The nine weeks are divided into three phases, each one lasting three weeks. I will give you guidelines regarding the number of sets and reps in each phase.

Why the different phases? Phasing your workout creates more effective workouts—in three ways. First, phasing allows you to "progressively overload" your body with harder and more challenging workouts.

Second, it changes the type of adaptation signal you send to your muscles. When you first start a workout, the stimulus is novel and new. This gets the body to adapt and change quickly, but as you continue the same exact type of workout, your body learns to become more efficient at it. The stimulus then loses its effectiveness, resulting in plateaus (or stalls) in progress. In my experience, it is most effective to switch to a different type of stimulus before the plateau happens. For most people this is at around the three-week mark.

Third, phasing helps you learn how to lift properly in different rep ranges. Low rep ranges require you to get tight, maintain stability, and summon maximal strength, whereas higher rep ranges require more strength endurance and stamina. Phasing also allows you to learn and maintain good form, proper breathing, and technique as your muscles fatigue and burn.

4. Pay attention to soreness. No soreness or a little soreness from a workout is fine. If you are sore to the touch or your soreness is felt every time you move or if the soreness lasts for longer than two days, you trained too hard or too long for your individual body. This will result in slower progress and fewer results. Try backing off the resistance slightly.

Follow these guidelines and you'll be resistance-ready. So, let's get started!

7

THE TOTAL BODY
ANYWHERE PROGRAM

Welcome to the Total Body Anywhere Program! If you're a beginner and brand-new to resistance training, this is the place to start.

One of the best parts of resistance training is that you can do it anywhere. Most of the time, it doesn't cost much, either, and doesn't take much time. You don't have to drive to the gym, or commit to a time slot. There's no expensive gym membership required either.

What's more, you can get fit and strong using only three pieces of equipment: resistance bands, a stability ball, and your own bodyweight. Use these tools pretty much anywhere—in your bedroom or basement or in a room away from home, at your office, while on vacation or taking a business trip.

I have found it to be extremely effective at getting people great results with proper nutrition and minimal workout time. It also builds consistency, which tends to lead to helping you eventually progress to spending more time working out and maybe even eventually joining a gym. It covers the whole body and works very well for a majority of people.

Follow it, and you'll get in shape in the short and long term.

THE ONLY THREE PIECES OF EQUIPMENT YOU NEED

Resistance Bands

Portable, affordable, and limitless in use, resistance bands are among the most overlooked pieces of fitness equipment. They take up very little space and are supereasy to travel with.

Resistance bands have been around in some form or another since the early twentieth century. In those early days, they were mostly used to help rehabilitate patients with damaged or weak muscles. The bands helped them recuperate their lost strength. Today, resistance bands are still used in the rehabilitation field, as well as by anyone looking to strengthen their muscles and create a more fit body.

Resistance bands are:

- Versatile because they let you target every part of your body
- Strength building because they can be used to make an exercise harder or easier, for upper body or lower body. The bands induce muscular contraction, which builds strength in your muscles as you pull against the band.
- Available in different resistance levels. Resistance bands are essentially thick, colorful elastic bands that come in a variety of shapes, thicknesses, and sizes. This allows you to progress with higher resistances as you build greater strength. I prefer bands that have handles; they are easier to work with.

If you are unsure which resistance band to buy, I recommend getting a full set of different resistances so that you can progress with the band, starting with a lighter resistance and progressing to a more challenging one.

In general, a thicker band gives you greater resistance. The color of the band is also an indicator. Typically, yellows and oranges are usually lightest, with reds and blues in the middle, and greens, purples, and blacks the most resistant.

If you perform an exercise that you haven't done before, practice it first without the band. This lets you get a feel for the proper movement without putting stress on your body. What you practice is what you get good at. Once you're comfortable with the exercise and confident in what you're doing, perform it with the resistance band.

Progress slowly to the bands with greater resistance. Go slowly and make sure you have mastered one band completely before you tackle the next level.

Stability Ball

The stability ball was invented in 1963 by an Italian plastics manufacturer who discovered the tool in Switzerland (which is why it is sometimes called a "Swiss ball"). Like resistance bands, the stability ball was originally used in physical therapy for rehabilitation. It entered the fitness world in the '80s, and despite falling in and out of favor at times, it has become an important piece of training equipment. It is useful for beginners, intermediate exercisers, and advanced exercisers.

In fact, in addition to barbells and dumbbells, it was the number one tool I used with my clients. It has many benefits. The stability ball:

- Teaches you be stable while working out, and to control your body
- Encourages perfect form while exercising. Proper form helps build strength and fitness.
- Strengthens your proprioceptive ability, which refers to your awareness of where your body is in space
- Develops core strength and sculpts your abs. The stability ball has many uses, but its number one application is in core training. Its spherical construction, for example, molds to your lumbar spine when you do crunches—a position that allows you to better activate your ab and core muscles. By contrast, some of the gym equipment for ab training can hurt your back. The stability ball does not.

There is tremendous value in using a stability ball. Be sure to have one in your home gym.

Your Own Bodyweight

You might not realize it, but you have at your disposal one of the best resistance training tools ever: your own bodyweight. Bodyweight workouts are extremely effective. A study published in the American College of Sports Medicine's *Health and Fitness Journal* found that bodyweight workouts are an efficient way to decrease body fat, improve VO_2max (your body's ability to process oxygen), and boost muscular fitness. Additionally, bodyweight training:

- Effectively works your muscles, improves your physique, and develops an athletic-looking body (like that of gymnasts who do primarily bodyweight training)
- Conditions your joints and keeps them strong
- Develops mobility, flexibility, and stability
- Improves coordination

Your body is your equipment! Because many bodyweight moves are performed on the floor, I suggest purchasing an exercise mat.

THE TOTAL BODY ANYWHERE EXERCISES

Before beginning the workouts, it's a good idea to read through these instructions and study the photographs. Then, be sure to practice the moves to get the feel of each exercise.

The Primers

CROSS LEG PRIMER

Start: Sit in a chair or on a bench with your knees bent at 90 degrees and both feet planted firmly on the ground. Place one foot on top of your other knee in a cross-legged position. Sit really tall with a straight back.

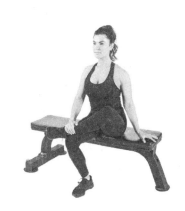

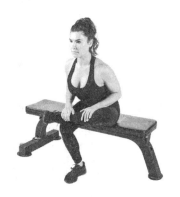

Action: If you can, try to lean forward a little while maintaining posture. While doing this (or attempting to do this), try to press the foot that is crossed into the leg it is resting on and try to bring the knee of the crossed leg down. Do this *only* using the strength of the crossed leg, without help from your hands. You will feel the leg muscles and the glute muscles of the crossed leg fire and burn. Hold this pressing position for 5 to 10 seconds, then rest for 10 to 20 seconds and repeat. After half of the recommended time is up, switch legs and repeat.

CHAIR COMBAT PRIMER

Start: Stand in front of a chair or bench with one foot on the chair and the other on the ground. Bring the knee of the leg that is on the chair as far forward as you can while keeping the foot that is on the floor totally flat.

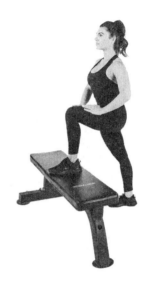

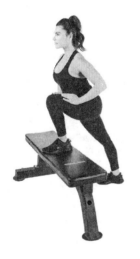

Action: Once you feel like your heel wants to raise and you can't move farther forward, hold that position and *try* to pull upward the toes of the foot that is on the chair. Don't worry when you can't pull your toes up; the point is to try. You should feel the muscles on your shin burn and fire. Hold this for 5 to 10 seconds, then back off and rest for 10 to 20 seconds. Do this until half of the recommended time is up, then repeat with the other leg.

FLOOR SHOULDER PRIMER

Start: Lie flat on your back with
your knees bent. Start with your
arms bent, with elbows, arms, and
back of hands touching floor.

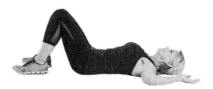

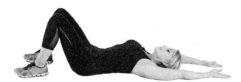

Action: Reach as if you are
trying to make your arms
longer while simultaneously
maintaining contact with the
floor with your entire arm.
Imagine you are making
yourself longer. Reach hard
for 5 to 10 seconds, then
back off and rest for 10 to
20 seconds. Do this until the
recommended time is up.

PRONE COBRA PRIMER

Start: Lie facedown on the floor or an exercise mat. Keep your arms out at your sides, as shown.

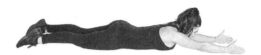

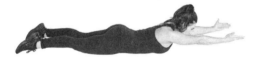

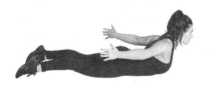

Action: Simultaneously, lift your chest, arms, and feet off the floor. Pull your arms back while retracting your shoulders. Squeeze your shoulder blades. Return to the starting position.

The Exercises

Workout 1

BODYWEIGHT SQUATS

Start: Stand with your feet about shoulder- to hip-width apart with your arms folded in front of your chest. Ideally, your feet should point forward, but you may angle them out slightly as well. Keep your core tight.

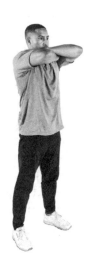

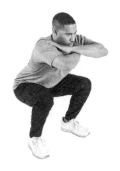

Action: Simultaneously bend your knees and slide your hips back. Raise and cross your arms and slightly fold your upper body forward. Keep sitting down until your thighs are parallel to the floor. You may take a deeper bend if your mobility allows it.

Straighten your knees and drive back up to the starting position, pushing back up off your feet. This completes one rep.

PUSH-UPS ON KNEES

Start: Assume the standard push-up position. Next, get down on your knees instead of placing your weight on your feet. Cross your feet behind you. Make sure your arms are straight with your hands shoulder-width apart on the floor or an exercise mat and palms placed down. Make sure your butt is not sticking up in their air. The alignment of your back should be at a perfect slant.

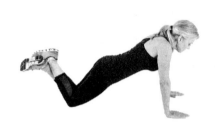

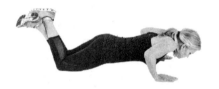

Action: Lower your chest to the floor by bending at the elbows. Don't let your hips droop down. Pause, then push back up to starting position. This completes one rep.

ALTERNATIVE: FULL PUSH-UPS

Start: Assume the standard push-up position. Position hands shoulder-width apart on the floor or an exercise mat. Your arms should be straight. Keep your core tight.

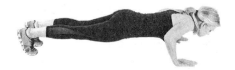

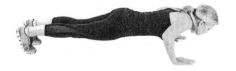

Action: Lower your chest to the floor by bending at the elbows. Don't let your hips droop down. Pause, then push back up to starting position. This completes one rep.

SEATED BAND ROWS

Start: Anchor your resistance band to a sturdy object. Sit on a bench or chair, or on the floor, as far as the band extends. Sit with an upright posture (straight back). Keep your core tight. Keep your feet flat on the floor. Grasp the handles with both hands.

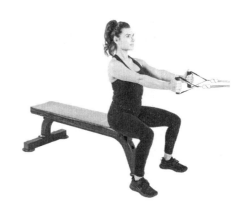

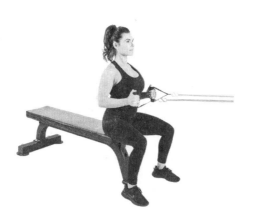

Action: Pull the band and handles in toward your midsection, and squeeze your shoulder blades back and down (imagine pinching a pencil between your shoulder blades). Keep your arms close to your body while pulling. Return to the starting position. This completes one rep.

OVERHEAD BAND PRESS

Start: Place one foot on the midpoint of the band, anchoring it to the floor. Grasp the handles, bend your elbows, and pull them up to chin-level, with your palms facing inward. Keep your elbows close to your ribs. Maintain a tight grasp on the handles to keep your wrists strong.

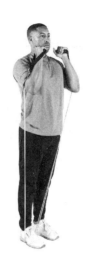

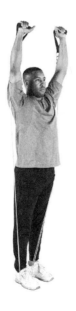

Action: Press upward with both hands through a full range of motion until you reach the starting position. This completes one rep.

HIP FLEXOR DEACTIVATOR CRUNCHES

Start: Lie flat on your back on the floor or an exercise mat, elevating your feet slightly on a bench or chair. Rotate your pelvis to flatten your back against the floor. Fold your arms over your chest.

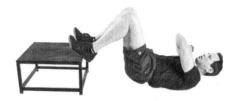

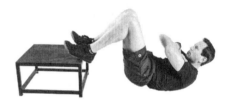

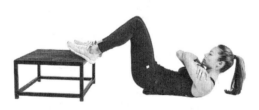

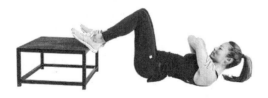

Action: Press your heels into the bench or chair, which should *slightly* lift your hips off the floor. You should feel your hamstrings and glutes firing. Crunch up from your sternum to your belly button, while contracting your abs. Your glutes should be engaged throughout the entire movement. Return to the starting position. This completes one rep.

BAND CHOP

Start: Anchor your resistance band to a sturdy and stable structure. Grip the handles with both hands and extend your elbows in front of your chest. Stand upright with proper posture.

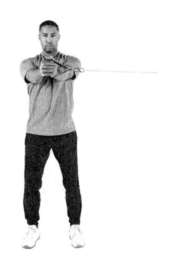

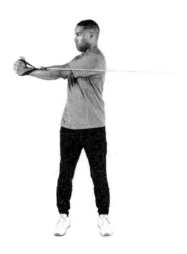

Action: Pull your arms and shoulders across your hips, rotating at your waist. Keep your hips from twisting, while maintaining a tight core. Rotate back to the starting position. This completes one rep.

Workout 2

EXTERNAL/INTERNAL HIP ROTATION ON CHAIR

Start: Place a bent knee on a bench or chair, preferably with a soft seat cushion.

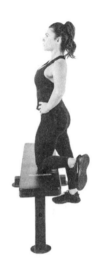

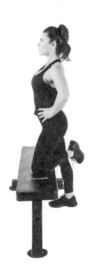

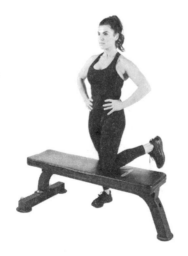

Action: While keeping your knee bent at 90 degrees, rotate your leg outward as far as you can and hold for 3 seconds, then inward as far as you can and hold for 3 seconds. Keep your hips and body as straight as possible. The body should not move, just the leg. This completes one rep. Do this until the recommended time is up.

SLOW ECCENTRIC CALF RAISE

Start: Stand up on the balls of your feet. (To make this exercise more challenging, stand on the edge of a stair or elevated platform, with your heels slightly overhanging the surface.)

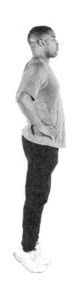

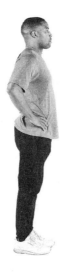

Action: Slowly lower your heels until you feel a stretch. When you get to the bottom, try to lift your toes as high as you can as if you are trying to get them to touch your shins. You won't be able to move much but this is okay; the intention is what is important. Pull toes up while your heels are at the bottom for 5 to 10 seconds, then step down and rest for 10 to 20 seconds. Repeat until time is up.

WALL PRESS

Start: Place your hips, lower back, upper back, and "occipital bun" (which feels like a bony nodule at the lower back part of your skull) flat against a wall, with your feet a comfortable distance apart. Place the back of your arms against the wall, as shown, but without shrugging your shoulders upward. Position your feet about a foot away from the wall.

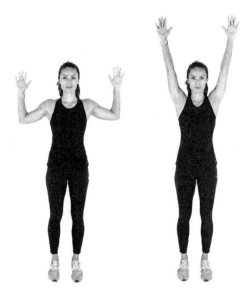

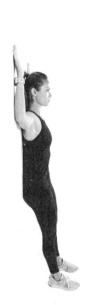

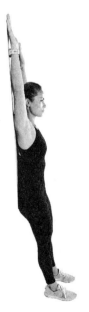

Action: Press all contact points (hips, upper back, lower back, and head) into the wall. Raise your arms overhead, as shown. Relax to the starting position. This completes one rep.

STATIONARY LUNGE

Start: Stand with your feet a comfortable distance apart. Place your hands on your hips. Keep your shoulders back and your chest up.

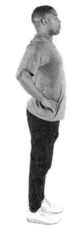

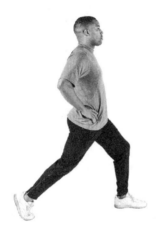

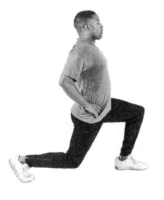

Action: Take a giant step forward while raising your back heel. Keep your chest up and squat down to a reasonable depth. Go up and down with your feet staying in position. Repeat with the opposite leg, then return to the starting position. This completes one rep.

PUSH-UP WITH HAND RELEASE

Start: Begin at the top of a traditional push-up position, with your hands on the ground slightly wider than shoulder width. You can perform this exercise on your knees, if you wish.

Make sure your body forms a straight line from your head to your feet. Keep your core tight.

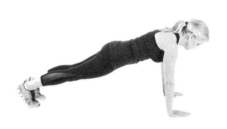

Action: Lower your body to the floor. Keep your elbows close to your sides. Once your chest is on the ground, release your hands from the floor and point your elbows toward the ceiling. Squeeze your shoulder blades together.

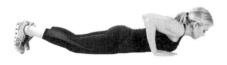

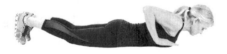

Place your hands back in the correct position and use the same form you came down with to push yourself back to the starting position. Keep your core tight and your body in a straight line. Return to the starting position. This completes one rep.

BAND PULL-APART

Start: With your feet a comfortable distance apart, bend your knees slightly. Grasp a length of the resistance band in both hands, as shown. Your hands should be slightly wider than shoulder-width apart. Extend your arms upward in front of you, at about shoulder level.

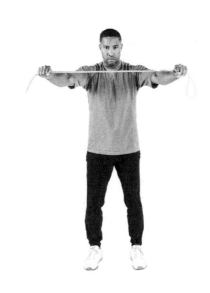

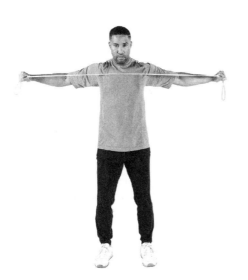

Action: With your core drawn in, stretch the band outward with both hands as far as you can. Try to keep your shoulders from elevating. Return to the starting position and repeat. This completes one rep.

BAND TRICEPS PRESSDOWN

Start: Anchor the middle part of your band to a sturdy overhead structure. Stand with your feet about 12 inches apart and bend your knees slightly. Grasp the handles of the resistance band, palms facing downward. Keep your upper arms bent and elbows tight against your upper body

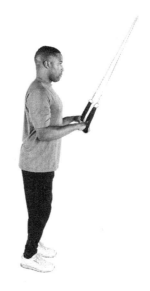

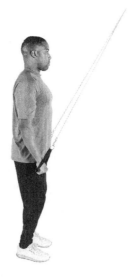

Action: Slowly extend arms down to full elbow lockout, feeling tension in your triceps muscles. Then, slowly return to the starting position. This completes one rep.

BAND BICEPS CURLS

Start: Step on the band, with your feet about 12 inches apart (the farther apart you place your feet, the greater the resistance). Grasp the handles of the resistance band, palms facing upward. Begin with your arms at your sides. Keep your core tight.

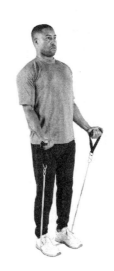

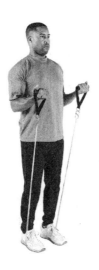

Action: Flex your elbows and curl upward until your hands meet your shoulders. Slowly lower to the starting position. This completes one rep.

BALL CRUNCH

Start: Sit on the ball with your feet flat on the floor and hip width apart. Roll back on the ball so that your mid- to lower back is in contact with the ball and your upper body is parallel to the floor. Place your hands near the sides of the head or cross your arms over your chest.

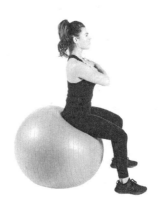

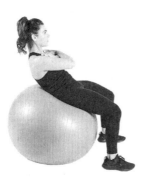

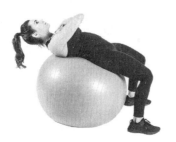

Action: Slowly curl up your upper body so that your upper back is off the ball. Uncurl your upper body. Press your hips up while crunching and keep them elevated the whole time. Return to the start position in a slow and controlled manner. This completes one rep.

The Total Body Anywhere Workout

With each exercise, perform the number of sets specified within the recommended rep range.

Exercises	Phase 1			Phase 2			Phase 3		
	Week 1	Week 2	Week 3	Week 4	Week 5	Week 6	Week 7	Week 8	Week 9
Workout 1 (Monday and optional Friday)									
Cross Leg Primer	1 minute	1 minute	1 minute	1 minute	1 minute	1 minute	1 minute	1 minute	1 minute
Chair Combat Primer	1 minute	1 minute	1 minute	1 minute	1 minute	1 minute	1 minute	1 minute	1 minute
Floor Shoulder Primer	1 minute	1 minute	1 minute	1 minute	1 minute	1 minute	1 minute	1 minute	1 minute
Prone Cobra Primer	1 minute	1 minute	1 minute	1 minute	1 minute	1 minute	1 minute	1 minute	1 minute
Bodyweight Squats	▪1 set ▪5 to 20 reps	▪1 set ▪5 to 20 reps	▪1 set ▪5 to 20 reps	▪2 sets ▪5 to 20 reps	▪2 sets ▪5 to 20 reps	▪2 sets ▪5 to 20 reps	▪3 sets ▪5 to 20 reps	▪3 sets ▪5 to 20 reps	▪3 sets ▪5 to 20 reps
Push-Ups on Knees or Full Push-Ups	▪1 set ▪5 to 20 reps	▪1 set ▪5 to 20 reps	▪1 set ▪5 to 20 reps	▪2 sets ▪5 to 20 reps	▪2 sets ▪5 to 20 reps	▪2 sets ▪5 to 20 reps	▪3 sets ▪5 to 20 reps	▪3 sets ▪5 to 20 reps	▪3 sets ▪5 to 20 reps
Seated Band Rows	▪1 set ▪5 to 20 reps	▪1 set ▪5 to 20 reps	▪1 set ▪5 to 20 reps	▪2 sets ▪5 to 20 reps	▪2 sets ▪5 to 20 reps	▪2 sets ▪5 to 20 reps	▪3 sets ▪5 to 20 reps	▪3 sets ▪5 to 20 reps	▪3 sets ▪5 to 20 reps
Overhead Band Press	▪1 set ▪5 to 20 reps	▪1 set ▪5 to 20 reps	▪1 set ▪5 to 20 reps	▪2 sets ▪5 to 20 reps	▪2 sets ▪5 to 20 reps	▪2 sets ▪5 to 20 reps	▪3 sets ▪5 to 20 reps	▪3 sets ▪5 to 20 reps	▪3 sets ▪5 to 20 reps
Hip Flexor Deactivator Crunches	▪1 set ▪5 to 20 reps	▪1 set ▪5 to 20 reps	▪1 set ▪5 to 20 reps	▪2 sets ▪5 to 20 reps	▪2 sets ▪5 to 20 reps	▪2 sets ▪5 to 20 reps	▪3 sets ▪5 to 20 reps	▪3 sets ▪5 to 20 reps	▪3 sets ▪5 to 20 reps
Band Chop	▪1 set ▪5 to 20 reps	▪1 set ▪5 to 20 reps	▪1 set ▪5 to 20 reps	▪2 sets ▪5 to 20 reps	▪2 sets ▪5 to 20 reps	▪2 sets ▪5 to 20 reps	▪3 sets ▪5 to 20 reps	▪3 sets ▪5 to 20 reps	▪3 sets ▪5 to 20 reps

continues

continued

Exercises	Phase 1			Phase 2			Phase 3		
	Week 1	Week 2	Week 3	Week 4	Week 5	Week 6	Week 7	Week 8	Week 9
Workout 2 (Wednesday)									
Prone Cobra Primer	1 minute	1 minute	1 minute	1 minute	1 minute	1 minute	1 minute	1 minute	1 minute
External/ Internal Hip Rotation on Chair	1 minute	1 minute	1 minute	1 minute	1 minute	1 minute	1 minute	1 minute	1 minute
Slow Eccentric Calf Raise	30 seconds	30 seconds	30 seconds	30 seconds	30 seconds	30 seconds	30 seconds	30 seconds	30 seconds
Wall Press	1 minute	1 minute	1 minute	1 minute	1 minute	1 minute	1 minute	1 minute	1 minute
Stationary Lunge	▪1 set ▪5 to 20 reps	▪1 set ▪5 to 20 reps	▪1 set ▪5 to 20 reps	▪2 sets ▪5 to 20 reps	▪2 sets ▪5 to 20 reps	▪2 sets ▪5 to 20 reps	▪3 sets ▪5 to 20 reps	▪3 sets ▪5 to 20 reps	▪3 sets ▪5 to 20 reps
Push-Up with Hand Release (knees or feet)	▪1 set ▪5 to 20 reps	▪1 set ▪5 to 20 reps	▪1 set ▪5 to 20 reps	▪2 sets ▪5 to 20 reps	▪2 sets ▪5 to 20 reps	▪2 sets ▪5 to 20 reps	▪3 sets ▪5 to 20 reps	▪3 sets ▪5 to 20 reps	▪3 sets ▪5 to 20 reps
Band Pull-Apart	▪1 set ▪5 to 20 reps	▪1 set ▪5 to 20 reps	▪1 set ▪5 to 20 reps	▪2 sets ▪5 to 20 reps	▪2 sets ▪5 to 20 reps	▪2 sets ▪5 to 20 reps	▪3 sets ▪5 to 20 reps	▪3 sets ▪5 to 20 reps	▪3 sets ▪5 to 20 reps
Band Triceps Pressdown	▪1 set ▪5 to 20 reps	▪1 set ▪5 to 20 reps	▪1 set ▪5 to 20 reps	▪2 sets ▪5 to 20 reps	▪2 sets ▪5 to 20 reps	▪2 sets ▪5 to 20 reps	▪3 sets ▪5 to 20 reps	▪3 sets ▪5 to 20 reps	▪3 sets ▪5 to 20 reps
Band Biceps Curls	▪1 set ▪5 to 20 reps	▪1 set ▪5 to 20 reps	▪1 set ▪5 to 20 reps	▪2 sets ▪5 to 20 reps	▪2 sets ▪5 to 20 reps	▪2 sets ▪5 to 20 reps	▪3 sets ▪5 to 20 reps	▪3 sets ▪5 to 20 reps	▪3 sets ▪5 to 20 reps
Ball Crunch	▪1 set ▪5 to 20 reps	▪1 set ▪5 to 20 reps	▪1 set ▪5 to 20 reps	▪2 sets ▪5 to 20 reps	▪2 sets ▪5 to 20 reps	▪2 sets ▪5 to 20 reps	▪3 sets ▪5 to 20 reps	▪3 sets ▪5 to 20 reps	▪3 sets ▪5 to 20 reps

THE MOBILITY PROGRAM

By now, you've heard me emphasize mobility quite a bit. And for good reason: it is the number one factor to consider as you pursue resistance training. Improving your mobility gives you lots of perks: improved ability to move with control with larger ranges of motion (which means you get better results from your exercises); healing from chronic pain in certain areas of your body; and the prevention of workout injuries.

Mobility-based movements are typically not the same as strength- or muscle-building movements. They usually don't require weights. There are many to choose from, and the ones you need to pick are those that work best for *you*.

The exercises all depend on which area of the body needs work. Okay, sounds simple enough. But please understand that usually body parts needing better mobility require some consistent time to improve. You have to keep doing mobility work.

For starters, I suggest you review Chapter 3 and look at the results of the mobility assessments you did there. They will pinpoint the areas to work on. This is important! Focusing on shoulder mobility every single day won't do you much good if it's your hip or ankle mobility that you need to work on.

Once you determine your areas of issue, work on them for ten to fifteen minutes every single day. Within a very short period of time you should see significant improvements in your mobility and overall fitness progress.

Several mobility exercises are already built into the previous workouts. Here are some of my favorite mobility movements for the most common target areas that people tend to need help with. Add the ones you need into any of the workouts in this book.

Mobility Exercises

Neck

NECK TRACTION ON THE WALL

Start: Stand with your shoulders, upper back, lower back, and hips pressed against the wall.

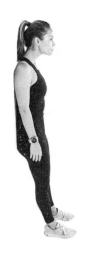

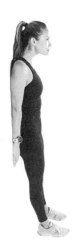
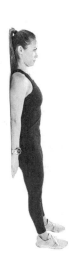

Action: While keeping everything in contact with wall, drive your shoulders down, followed by your lower back and head against the wall. Try to elongate your neck for 10 seconds. Repeat 5 times.

ROTATION WITH TENSION

Start: Stand with your shoulders, upper back, lower back, and hips pressed against the wall.

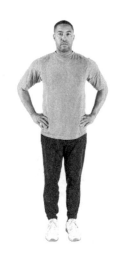

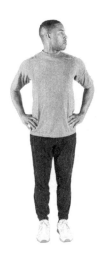

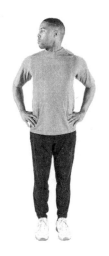

Action: While keeping everything in contact with wall, drive your shoulders down, followed by your lower back and head against the wall. Try to elongate your neck.

Maintain the contact points against wall. Slowly turn your head as far left as you can; then turn your head to the right as far as you can. Do these moves slowly for 10 total reps (5 to the left and 5 to the right).

Upper Back and Shoulders

Handcuff with Rotation (see page 157)
Prone Cobra Primer (see page 116)

Lower Back

CAT AND COW

Start: Get down on your hands and knees on the floor or an exercise mat.

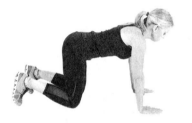

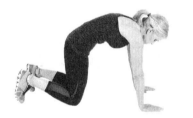

Action: Round your back as much as possible while looking down and exhaling. Then, arch your back, dropping your belly toward the floor and looking up while inhaling. Repeat 5 to 10 times.

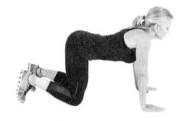

Pelvic Tilts (see page 158)

Hips

Frogger (see page 156)

Ankles and Feet

Combat Stretch (see page 146)

SHORT FOOT

Start: You can perform
this exercise in a sitting or
standing position.

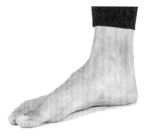

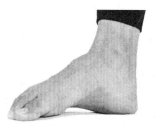

Action: Create an arch in
your foot by squeezing the
foot "shorter," as shown.
Squeeze and hold for 5
seconds. Repeat 5 to 10
times on each foot.

Hands and Wrist

WRIST EXTENSION

Start: Stand with your feet a comfortable distance apart. Extend both arms out in front of you, palms up. Then flex your wrists downward, as shown.

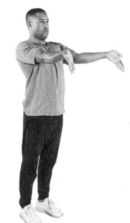

Action: While maintaining the start position, begin to rock your body forward. Do 5 to 10 slow reps for 3 sets.

WRIST FLEXION

Start: Stand with your feet a comfortable distance apart. Extend both arms out in front of you, palms down. Then flex your wrists downward so that your fingers are pointing toward the floor, as shown.

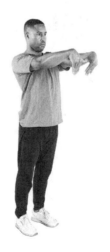

Action: While maintaining the start position, begin to rock your body back. Do 5 to 10 slow reps for 3 sets.

WHAT ABOUT MOBILITY MOVES FOR THE KNEE?

In my experience, chronic knee pain that isn't due to actual structural damage or injury (not an acute injury) is almost always caused by poor movement patterns and mobility issues in the hips, ankles, and feet.

The knee bends in one direction; meanwhile, the hips, ankles, and feet can rotate and bend in many different directions. If your hips and ankles are lacking in mobility in any direction or they lack strength and stability, your knees suffer the biggest consequences. Thus, fixing mobility issues in the hips, ankles, and feet helps tremendously if you have common chronic knee pain.

TAKE IT ON THE ROAD!

Travel can be an absolute nightmare for any fitness-minded person. Nothing will halt your muscle gain, fat loss, or athletic performance progress like interrupting a successful workout routine with a new time zone, a break in workouts, or airport and hotel food. It was one of the hardest challenges I helped my executive professional clients tackle when I was a personal trainer.

A good plan before travel that is implemented properly will keep your body on track in terms of your fitness goals. I have even had clients progress *faster* from a well-programmed travel workout plan due to the change in exercise stimulus.

No joke, travel does not have to mean your fitness has to take a backseat to your business success. In fact, according to some of my most successful executive professional clients, they found that they performed better in their business meetings and sales presentations when they followed my travel workout plans and adhered to my dietary and sleep advice. So, pack your resistance bands, do the Total Body Anywhere Program properly, and not only will you be more fit with more muscle, less fat, and better fitness, but you will also do better in business.

8

THE TOTAL BODY DUMBBELL PROGRAM

The dumbbell is probably the single most versatile tool for resistance training ever invented. Dumbbells can train any body part. They can be employed by anyone, regardless of training level or fitness experience. And they can be used in home gyms, regular gyms, and on the road.

Dumbbells have been with us for more than two thousand years, making them the oldest continuously used piece of exercise equipment ever. They date back to the ancient Greeks in the fifth century, who used them to perform exercises familiar to us today: biceps curls and lunges.

So, with only a set of dumbbells, you can get an effective, solid workout—one that develops strength and fitness in your upper and lower body. It is a workout that does it all.

The two workouts here provide a good number of exercises to work and sculpt your muscles, and like all the workouts here, they should not take longer than thirty to forty-five minutes.

Most of the exercises are "compound movements," meaning they activate multiple muscle groups across more than one joint. Compound movements are superchallenging to your body, and they get results. This workout also includes a variety of movement patterns, such as squatting, pushing, pulling, and more. This benefit helps you not only get stronger and fitter but also helps you move through your daily life easier and more comfortably.

All you need for these workouts is a set of dumbbells that come in different poundages. That way, you can increase your resistance and keep your muscles in adaptation mode.

I suggest purchasing one set of medium to heavy dumbbells for your lower-body exercises and one set of light to medium dumbbells for the upper-body moves. Alternatively, you can buy adjustable dumbbells, which let you change the weight according to your progress.

Once you get started, your entire body will be feeling these workouts.

The Exercises

Workout 1

90/90 PRIMER

Start: Sit on the floor or an exercise mat, with your legs angled out. Lean to one side, and slide your legs to move into a 90-degree angle. Keep your back knee in line with your shoulder. Tighten your glutes and core to prop up your upper body. Maintain a tall upright posture.

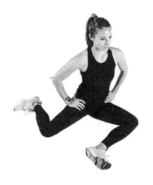

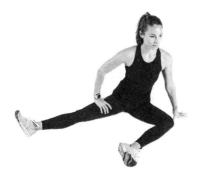

Action: Move into a 90/90 position, as shown, without hand support. Return to the start position. Do 30 seconds with one leg in front, then switch to the other leg for a total of 1 minute.

COMBAT STRETCH

Start: This stretch is performed near the corner of a wall. Begin in a kneeling position, as shown. Place the bended leg close to the wall. Turn your back foot out toward the bent leg. Place your hands on your hips.

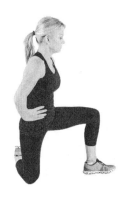

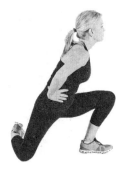

Action: Press your hips forward and lean forward, driving your forward knee toward your toes. Keep your knee from touching the wall. Once you reach that point, actively pull your toes on your back foot toward your shin and hold. Continue this movement for 1 minute.

FLOOR ANGELS

Start: Lie on the floor or an exercise mat with your knees bent. Press your back firmly on the floor, and place your arms at your sides and your palms facing up.

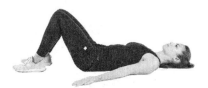

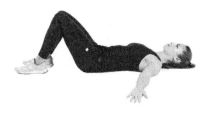

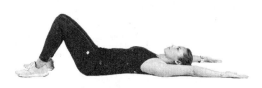

Action: With your elbows pressed on the floor, extend your arms and try to touch them over your head. Keep your elbows and wrists in contact with the floor throughout the entire range of motion. Continue this movement for 1 minute.

SINGLE LEG TOE TOUCH

Start: Begin with an upright posture. Stand with your feet about 12 inches apart, or at a comfortable distance. Raise your arms out to your sides, palms facing forward.

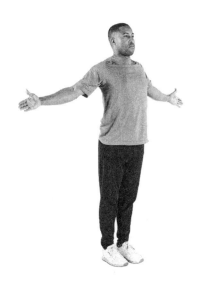

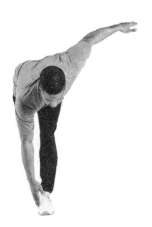

Action: Tense your core and lift one leg up behind you. Point your toe and flex your standing leg slightly for greater control. Reach with the opposite arm down to touch your toes. Repeat with the opposite leg. This completes one rep.

GOBLET SQUAT

Start: Hold one dumbbell by its head and place it in front of your chest, with your elbows tight against your body. Keep your shoulders back and your feet shoulder-width apart.

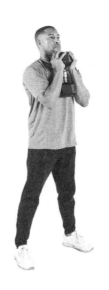

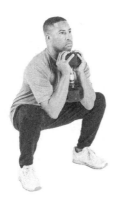

Action: Bend your knees and squat down as far as you can, keeping your arms inside your legs as you descend. Keep your hips and back rigid. Raise back up. This completes one rep.

DUMBBELL ROW

Start: Place your left knee on a bench, as shown, with your right leg on the floor. Grasp a dumbbell in your right hand. Pin your shoulders back with the dumbbell at midthigh. Keep your chest high and hinge forward at your hips until you reach a 45-degree angle to the floor. Tighten your core to support your back.

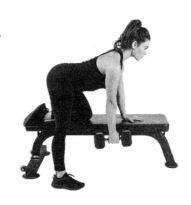

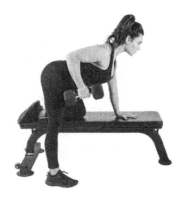

Action: Pull the weight upward to about chest level and squeeze your shoulder blades together at the top of the movement. Lower the dumbbell back down to the starting position. This completes one rep.

CHEST PRESS

Start: Lie on your back on your bench. Grasp a dumbbell in each hand. Begin with your elbows bent and the dumbbells held at chest-level. Brace your core and drive your feet into the floor for support.

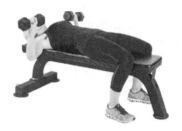

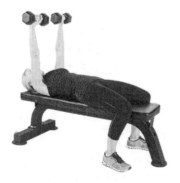

Action: Press the weights upward through a full range of motion. Lower slowly to the start position. This completes one rep.

DUMBBELL OVERHEAD PRESS

Start: Grasp a dumbbell
in each hand at your
shoulders with an
overhand grip. Your
thumbs should be on the
inside and knuckles facing
up. Stand upright and
keep your back straight.

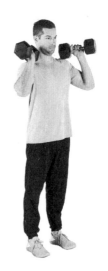

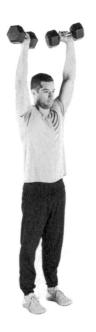

Action: Raise the weights
above your head in a
controlled motion and
pause at the top. Return
the dumbbells to the start
position. This completes
one rep.

Note: While the standing overhead press is a classic
move, you can perform the identical move while seated.
A seated dumbbell overhead press is a better option if
you are new to resistance training or if you have back
issues or injuries. To perform the exercise, simply sit on
a bench and follow the same steps.

HAMMER CURLS

Start: Stand with your feet a comfortable distance apart. Grasp a dumbbell in each hand and hold them at your sides. Stand with your shoulders back and down, your chest tall and your knees slightly bent.

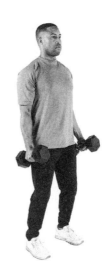

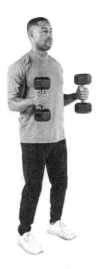

Action: With the weight-end of the dumbbells pointed toward the floor, curl up both dumbbells. Get a full range of motion with each set, while keeping your elbows close to your sides.

OVERHEAD TRICEPS PRESS

Start: Grasp a dumbbell in each hand. Tighten your core and angle one leg back slightly for support. Extend your arms above and behind your head.

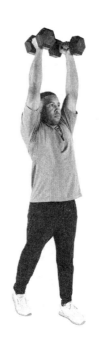

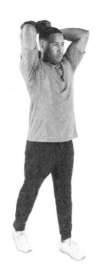

Action: Bend your elbows slightly and lower the weights behind your neck. Then, extend your elbows to straighten your arms against the resistance. This completes one rep. When you lower the weight, your elbows should point directly to the ceiling; do not let them shift forward or flare out to the side.

SLOW CRUNCHES

Start: This exercise is a basic crunch; however, it should take about 10 seconds to complete and therefore is performed very slowly. Lie down on your back on the floor or an exercise mat. Plant your feet on the floor, hip-width apart, and your knees bent. Place your hands behind your head. Contract your ab muscles.

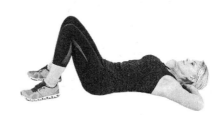

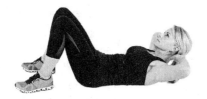

Action: Slowly lift your upper body toward your knees, keeping your head and neck relaxed. Slowly return to the starting position. This completes one 10-second rep.

Workout 2

FROGGER

Start: Lower your body to the floor. Brace yourself with your hands on the floor below your shoulders. Turn your legs and feet outward and press the inside of your feet and heels against the floor.

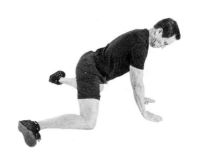

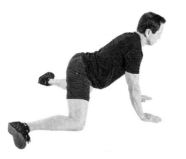

Action: Push your hips back as far as you can. Then, reverse the move and push all the way forward. Continue to move forward and back. You'll find your mobility improving the more you do this exercise.

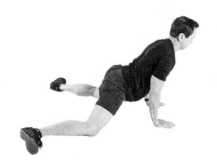

HANDCUFF WITH ROTATION

Start: Lie with your stomach on the floor or an exercise mat. Place the back of both hands together in the small of your back (as if you were handcuffed). Reach down with your arms, then out to your sides keeping your arms away from the floor. Slowly reach around then up above your head and as you do rotate your palms so that they face up toward the ceiling. Once they are straight up above your headband your elbows and touch the back of your neck. Keep going up and down in a slow and controlled motion.

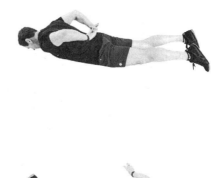

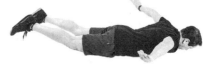

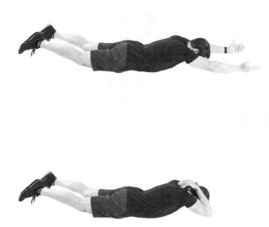

Action: Lower that arm so that your elbow touches the floor. Then, bring your arm back upward so that your elbow points to the ceiling. Keep going down and up, keeping your hand in the small of your back. Maintain a slow and controlled movement throughout the exercise, while exaggerating the stretch with each rotation. Repeat the exercise on the other side.

PELVIC TILTS

Start: Lie on your back with your knees bent. Keep your arms out at your sides, with palms facing upward and pressed against the floor. Your chin should be tucked.

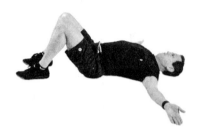

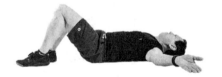

Action: Rotate your pelvis so that you have an arch in your lower back. Your hips should stay on the floor the whole time. Then, lower your pelvis back to the floor. Continue this tilting motion for 1 minute.

SUMO DEADLIFT

Start: Stand with your feet wider than shoulder-width apart. Point your toes outward. Grasp a dumbbell in each hand and hold them in front of your body, as shown.

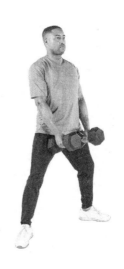

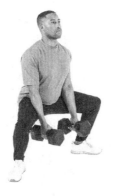

Action: Tighten your core. Keep your chest and head up, and lower your hips. Lift the dumbbells by straightening your legs and standing up straight. Make sure to keep your weight on your heels and bend through your hips and knees. This completes one rep.

DUMBBELL PULL-OVER

Start: Grasp a dumbbell with both hands, as shown, and lie with your back flat on a bench.

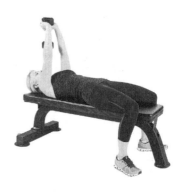

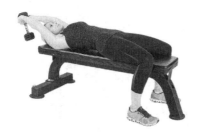

Action: With your feet planted on the floor and your core tight, extend your arms to the ceiling. Cup the dumbbell with both hands above your chest. Slowly bend your elbows to the point at which your biceps reach your ears. Slowly bring your arms back to above your chest. This completes one rep.

CHEST PRESS—ELBOWS IN

Start: Grasp a dumbbell in each hand. Lie on your back on a bench with your shoulders pinned down and back. Place your feet on the floor and squeeze your hips and legs. Keep your elbows in and close to your sides through the movement.

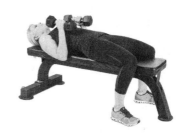

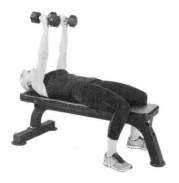

Action: Press the weights upward through a full range of motion, while maintaining a natural curve in your lower back. Lower the dumbbells to the start position. This completes one rep.

LATERAL RAISE

Start: Grasp a dumbbell in each hand and hold them at your sides. Stand with your feet about 12 inches apart. Keep your shoulders back and down and your chest tall. Tighten and brace your core through the entire exercise to prevent momentum.

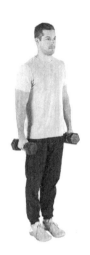

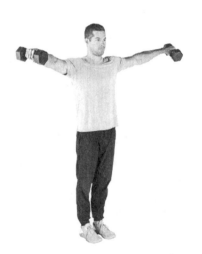

Action: Raise your arms to shoulder length, while keeping your elbows slightly bent. Keep your hips from hinging back. Lower back to the start position. This completes one rep.

SUPINATING CURLS

Start: Grasp a dumbbell in each hand so that your wrists are facing behind you. Stand with your feet a comfortable distance apart. Brace your core and maintain good posture for support. Keep your arms close to your body.

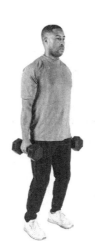

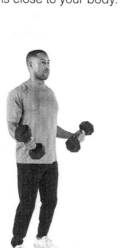

Action: Curl the weight toward your chest and shoulders, while externally rotating your forearm so that your wrist is facing toward you at the end of the curl. Lower back to start. This completes one rep.

BENCH DIP

Start: Sit down on a bench, your palms on the edge of the bench, fingers forward and next to your thighs. (You can also perform a bench dip off a stair, chair, or other elevated surface; the same steps apply.)

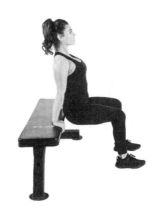

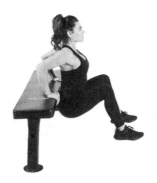

Action: Walk your feet slightly out, extending your legs. Lift your bottom off the bench and hold that position with your arms extended. Keep your bottom and back close to the bench. The farther out your feet are, the more difficult the exercise.

Hinging at your elbows, lower your body down as far as you can go, or until your arms form a 90-degree angle. Try to move through a full range of motion. Push up through your palms back to the starting position. This completes one rep.

PLANK

Start: Begin on your elbows and knees, as shown. Place your hands, forearms, and elbows under your shoulders on the floor or an exercise mat.

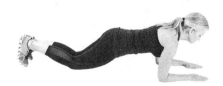

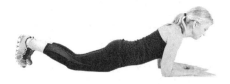

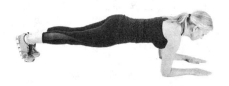

Action: Brace your core and extend your legs back and press your hips up. Tuck your tailbone forward, squeezing your abs. Hold the position for the specified amount of time.

THE ROUTINE

In this workout, choose whether to perform one to three sets for each phase. Base your selection on how you feel, how much time you have, and how sore you are from your previous workouts. This routine is phased by reps; you increase the number of reps you perform from phase to phase.

Exercises	Phase 1			Phase 2			Phase 3		
	Week 1	Week 2	Week 3	Week 4	Week 5	Week 6	Week 7	Week 8	Week 9
Workout 1 (Monday and optional Friday)									
90/90 Primer	1 minute	1 minute	1 minute	1 minute	1 minute	1 minute	1 minute	1 minute	1 minute
Combat Stretch	1 minute	1 minute	1 minute	1 minute	1 minute	1 minute	1 minute	1 minute	1 minute
Floor Angels	1 minute	1 minute	1 minute	1 minute	1 minute	1 minute	1 minute	1 minute	1 minute
Single Leg Toe Touch	▪1 to 3 sets ▪6 to 8 reps	▪1 to 3 sets ▪6 to 8 reps	▪1 to 3 sets ▪6 to 8 reps	▪1 to 3 sets ▪10 to 12 reps	▪1 to 3 sets ▪10 to 12 reps	▪1 to 3 sets ▪10 to 12 reps	▪1 to 3 sets ▪15 to 20 reps	▪1 to 3 sets ▪15 to 20 reps	▪1 to 3 sets ▪15 to 20 reps
Goblet Squat	▪1 to 3 sets ▪6 to 8 reps	▪1 to 3 sets ▪6 to 8 reps	▪1 to 3 sets ▪6 to 8 reps	▪1 to 3 sets ▪10 to 12 reps	▪1 to 3 sets ▪10 to 12 reps	▪1 to 3 sets ▪10 to 12 reps	▪1 to 3 sets ▪15 to 20 reps	▪1 to 3 sets ▪15 to 20 reps	▪1 to 3 sets ▪15 to 20 reps
Dumbbell Row	▪1 to 3 sets ▪6 to 8 reps	▪1 to 3 sets ▪6 to 8 reps	▪1 to 3 sets ▪6 to 8 reps	▪1 to 3 sets ▪10 to 12 reps	▪1 to 3 sets ▪10 to 12 reps	▪1 to 3 sets ▪10 to 12 reps	▪1 to 3 sets ▪15 to 20 reps	▪1 to 3 sets ▪15 to 20 reps	▪1 to 3 sets ▪15 to 20 reps
Chest Press	▪1 to 3 sets ▪6 to 8 reps	▪1 to 3 sets ▪6 to 8 reps	▪1 to 3 sets ▪6 to 8 reps	▪1 to 3 sets ▪10 to 12 reps	▪1 to 3 sets ▪10 to 12 reps	▪1 to 3 sets ▪10 to 12 reps	▪1 to 3 sets ▪15 to 20 reps	▪1 to 3 sets ▪15 to 20 reps	▪1 to 3 sets ▪15 to 20 reps
Dumbbell Overhead Press	▪1 to 3 sets ▪6 to 8 reps	▪1 to 3 sets ▪6 to 8 reps	▪1 to 3 sets ▪6 to 8 reps	▪1 to 3 sets ▪10 to 12 reps	▪1 to 3 sets ▪10 to 12 reps	▪1 to 3 sets ▪10 to 12 reps	▪1 to 3 sets ▪15 to 20 reps	▪1 to 3 sets ▪15 to 20 reps	▪1 to 3 sets ▪15 to 20 reps

continues

continued

Exercises	Phase 1			Phase 2			Phase 3		
	Week 1	Week 2	Week 3	Week 4	Week 5	Week 6	Week 7	Week 8	Week 9
Hammer Curls	▪ 1 to 3 sets ▪ 6 to 8 reps	▪ 1 to 3 sets ▪ 6 to 8 reps	▪ 1 to 3 sets ▪ 6 to 8 reps	▪ 1 to 3 sets ▪ 10 to 12 reps	▪ 1 to 3 sets ▪ 10 to 12 reps	▪ 1 to 3 sets ▪ 10 to 12 reps	▪ 1 to 3 sets ▪ 15 to 20 reps	▪ 1 to 3 sets ▪ 15 to 20 reps	▪ 1 to 3 sets ▪ 15 to 20 reps
Overhead Triceps Press	▪ 1 to 3 sets ▪ 6 to 8 reps	▪ 1 to 3 sets ▪ 6 to 8 reps	▪ 1 to 3 sets ▪ 6 to 8 reps	▪ 1 to 3 sets ▪ 10 to 12 reps	▪ 1 to 3 sets ▪ 10 to 12 reps	▪ 1 to 3 sets ▪ 10 to 12 reps	▪ 1 to 3 sets ▪ 15 to 20 reps	▪ 1 to 3 sets ▪ 15 to 20 reps	▪ 1 to 3 sets ▪ 15 to 20 reps
Slow Crunches	▪ 1 to 3 sets ▪ 6 to 8 reps	▪ 1 to 3 sets ▪ 6 to 8 reps	▪ 1 to 3 sets ▪ 6 to 8 reps	▪ 1 to 3 sets ▪ 10 to 12 reps	▪ 1 to 3 sets ▪ 10 to 12 reps	▪ 1 to 3 sets ▪ 10 to 12 reps	▪ 1 to 3 sets ▪ 15 to 20 reps	▪ 1 to 3 sets ▪ 15 to 20 reps	▪ 1 to 3 sets ▪ 15 to 20 reps
Workout 2 (Wednesday)									
Frogger	1 minute	1 minute	1 minute	1 minute	1 minute	1 minute	1 minute	1 minute	1 minute
Handcuff with Rotation	1 minute	1 minute	1 minute	1 minute	1 minute	1 minute	1 minute	1 minute	1 minute
Pelvic Tilts	1 minute	1 minute	1 minute	1 minute	1 minute	1 minute	1 minute	1 minute	1 minute
Single Leg Toe Touch	▪ 1 to 3 sets ▪ 6 to 8 reps	▪ 1 to 3 sets ▪ 6 to 8 reps	▪ 1 to 3 sets ▪ 6 to 8 reps	▪ 1 to 3 sets ▪ 10 to 12 reps	▪ 1 to 3 sets ▪ 10 to 12 reps	▪ 1 to 3 sets ▪ 10 to 12 reps	▪ 1 to 3 sets ▪ 15 to 20 reps	▪ 1 to 3 sets ▪ 15 to 20 reps	▪ 1 to 3 sets ▪ 15 to 20 reps
Sumo Deadlift	▪ 1 to 3 sets ▪ 6 to 8 reps	▪ 1 to 3 sets ▪ 6 to 8 reps	▪ 1 to 3 sets ▪ 6 to 8 reps	▪ 1 to 3 sets ▪ 10 to 12 reps	▪ 1 to 3 sets ▪ 10 to 12 reps	▪ 1 to 3 sets ▪ 10 to 12 reps	▪ 1 to 3 sets ▪ 15 to 20 reps	▪ 1 to 3 sets ▪ 15 to 20 reps	▪ 1 to 3 sets ▪ 15 to 20 reps
Dumbbell Pull-Over	▪ 1 to 3 sets ▪ 6 to 8 reps	▪ 1 to 3 sets ▪ 6 to 8 reps	▪ 1 to 3 sets ▪ 6 to 8 reps	▪ 1 to 3 sets ▪ 10 to 12 reps	▪ 1 to 3 sets ▪ 10 to 12 reps	▪ 1 to 3 sets ▪ 10 to 12 reps	▪ 1 to 3 sets ▪ 15 to 20 reps	▪ 1 to 3 sets ▪ 15 to 20 reps	▪ 1 to 3 sets ▪ 15 to 20 reps
Chest Press— Elbows In	▪ 1 to 3 sets ▪ 6 to 8 reps	▪ 1 to 3 sets ▪ 6 to 8 reps	▪ 1 to 3 sets ▪ 6 to 8 reps	▪ 1 to 3 sets ▪ 10 to 12 reps	▪ 1 to 3 sets ▪ 10 to 12 reps	▪ 1 to 3 sets ▪ 10 to 12 reps	▪ 1 to 3 sets ▪ 15 to 20 reps	▪ 1 to 3 sets ▪ 15 to 20 reps	▪ 1 to 3 sets ▪ 15 to 20 reps

continues

continued

Exercises	Phase 1			Phase 2			Phase 3		
	Week 1	Week 2	Week 3	Week 4	Week 5	Week 6	Week 7	Week 8	Week 9
Lateral Raise	▪1 to 3 sets ▪6 to 8 reps	▪1 to 3 sets ▪6 to 8 reps	▪1 to 3 sets ▪6 to 8 reps	▪1 to 3 sets ▪10 to 12 reps	▪1 to 3 sets ▪10 to 12 reps	▪1 to 3 sets ▪10 to 12 reps	▪1 to 3 sets ▪15 to 20 reps	▪1 to 3 sets ▪15 to 20 reps	▪1 to 3 sets ▪15 to 20 reps
Supinating Curls	▪1 to 3 sets ▪6 to 8 reps	▪1 to 3 sets ▪6 to 8 reps	▪1 to 3 sets ▪6 to 8 reps	▪1 to 3 sets ▪10 to 12 reps	▪1 to 3 sets ▪10 to 12 reps	▪1 to 3 sets ▪10 to 12 reps	▪1 to 3 sets ▪15 to 20 reps	▪1 to 3 sets ▪15 to 20 reps	▪1 to 3 sets ▪15 to 20 reps
Bench Dip	▪1 to 3 sets ▪6 to 8 reps	▪1 to 3 sets ▪6 to 8 reps	▪1 to 3 sets ▪6 to 8 reps	▪1 to 3 sets ▪10 to 12 reps	▪1 to 3 sets ▪10 to 12 reps	▪1 to 3 sets ▪10 to 12 reps	▪1 to 3 sets ▪15 to 20 reps	▪1 to 3 sets ▪15 to 20 reps	▪1 to 3 sets ▪15 to 20 reps
Plank	▪1 hold	▪1 hold	▪1 hold	▪2 holds	▪2 holds	▪2 holds	▪3 holds	▪3 holds	▪3 holds

9

THE TOTAL BODY FULL HOME GYM PROGRAM

Most at-home workouts end up being nothing more than long cardio sessions of walking or jogging on a treadmill or riding a stationary bike. They're good for burning some calories in the short term, but as I've emphasized, there isn't much value for strength building and fat burning—or for your metabolism. Obviously, if you can build an at-home gym setup with key pieces of resistance training equipment, that's a totally different story.

With this program, all you'll need is a set of barbells, an adjustable flat bench, a set of dumbbells, and a squat rack. If you've already invested in a stability ball and resistance bands, that's even better.

These tools allow you to perform the top best exercises for every body part. They include barbell squats, deadlifts, bench presses, shoulder presses, rows, barbell curls, and triceps extensions. Hands down, they are the best muscle and strength builders that exist. Because of their strength-building power, they are also amazing metabolism boosters and fat burners.

The best way to get in shape is to progress. So, if you have been doing my resistance band or dumbbell workouts for nine weeks, it's time to step up to this program for further muscle adaptation.

What this workout is also good at is getting you superaware of how your body moves and creating strong proprioception of being able to handle and control your bodyweight. This is important because a lot of injuries happen in the gym from people "ego lifting," showing off in the gym by lifting too much weight and taking it through a shortened range of motion in which they get very little effect. Being at home lets you focus on quality movement patterns and recognize your limitations and get better at them. Increasing your strength by taking your muscles through a proper, full range of motion is key here.

Also, in 2020, gyms had to close, and many of them went out of business due to Covid-19. If you were a gym-goer then, you probably wondered how you would keep your muscle, or make any further progress. Let me reassure you: this at-home workout can build a great physique and allow you to continue your fitness gains.

RAMP UP YOUR NEAT

NEAT stands for "nonexercise activity thermogenesis." Nonexercise is everything you do outside of your structured workout plan—walking through a parking lot, taking the stairs, and standing up at your desk—while thermogenesis is a fancy scientific term for the burning of calories.

Paying attention to NEAT is great for your health and fitness. According to a review study published in *Mayo Clinic Proceedings* in 2015, engaging more often in continuous, vital movements, such as fidgeting and standing—in other words, NEAT, can increase your daily calorie burn and prevent unhealthy weight gain.

So, how can you ramp up your NEAT? Some suggestions:

- Do more lifestyle activities, such as take the stairs, play with your kids, shovel snow, ride your bike, walk your dog, park farther away from buildings, rake leaves, and other activities.
- Stand more than you sit. Standing burns around 50 percent more calories than sitting—so stand up during TV commercials, during meetings, while talking on the phone, or sorting mail.
- Set your home and workplace up to promote more activity. Move your trash can and other essential items beyond an arm's reach away, for example.
- During breaks at work, walk the hallways or climb stairways.
- Turn mundane tasks into NEAT. While at the grocery store, do toe raises while waiting in line or walk some extra aisles.

Small changes through NEAT can lead to big changes over time.

The Exercises

Workout 1

90/90 Primer (see page 145)
Combat Stretch (see page 146)

WINDMILL

Start: Stand with your feet slightly wider than shoulder-width apart. Extend one arm straight up, with your other arm pointed downward. Keep your legs straight.

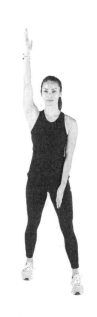

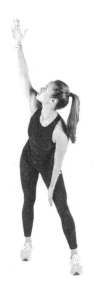

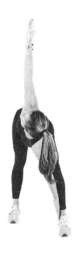

Start: Stand with your feet slightly wider than shoulder-width apart. Extend your right arm upward and keep your left arm straight down, as shown. Keep your legs straight.

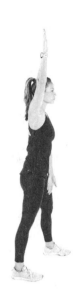

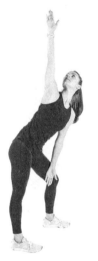

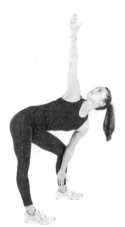

Action: Hinge at your hips and rotate your waist so that your left hand reaches down to touch your left foot.

Stand back up. Repeat the same motion, except this time bring your right hand down to touch your right foot. Stand back up again. Continue this rotating movement for 1 minute.

BOX/BENCH SQUATS

Start: Unrack the barbell and place it across the back of your shoulders. Stand in front of a sturdy box or bench. The bench height should place you at a parallel squat when you sit on it.

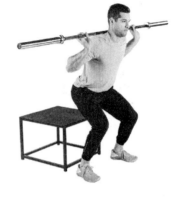

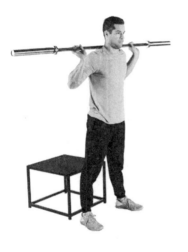

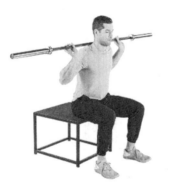

Action: Bend your knees, completely sit on the box, and straighten your back. Keep every muscle tight. To reverse the movement, drive upward off the box while maintaining a neutral spine. Squeeze your glutes at the top to finish. This completes one rep.

BARBELL SQUATS

Start: Place the barbell across the back of your shoulders when you are standing upright. Lift the bar up and walk out of the squat rack. Hold on to the bar with a firm grip, tensing and retracting your shoulders.

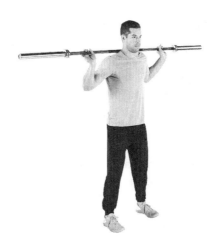

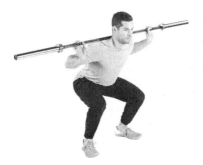

Action: Simultaneously bend your knees and slide your hips back and down. Drop into a full squat. Return to the starting position. This completes one rep.

BARBELL BENCH PRESS

Start: Lie on your back on the exercise bench. Grasp the barbell with your hands slightly wider than shoulder-width apart, as shown, and hold it across your upper chest. Keep your feet firmly planted on the floor. Draw in your core completely.

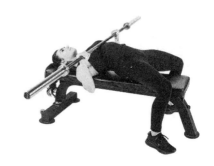

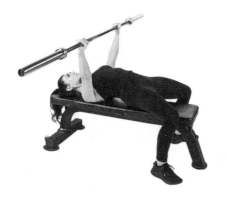

Action: Press the barbell upward. Then lower slowly to the start position, moving through a full range of motion. This completes one rep.

BARBELL ROW

Start: Stand with your feet about shoulder-width apart. Take a firm overhand grip on the barbell and hold it at the top of your thighs, as shown.

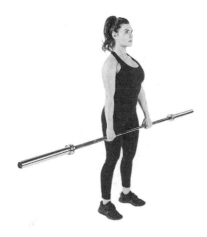

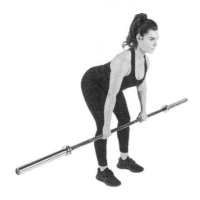

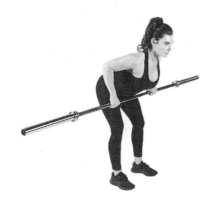

Action: Hinge your hips back with a slight bend in your knees. Lean forward slightly so that you are at a 45-degree angle to the floor. Keep your arms close to your sides and retract your shoulders as you pull the bar in toward your midsection. Then, straighten your arms as you lower the weight. This completes one rep. Move through a full range of motion as you execute this "rowing" motion.

BARBELL OVERHEAD PRESS

Start: Grasp a barbell using an overhand grip, with your hands slightly wider than shoulder-width apart. Stand up straight with your feet about hip-width apart. Bring the bar up to just below your chin, with your palms facing forward.

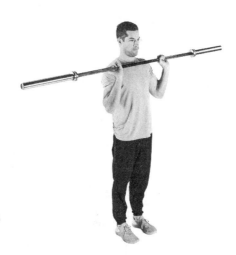

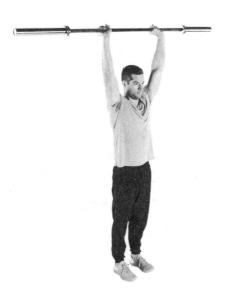

Action: Press the bar overhead until your arms are extended. Slowly return to the starting position, moving through a complete range of motion. This completes one rep.

Note: This exercise can be performed while seated on a bench.

BARBELL CURLS

Start: Place the barbell in front of you on the floor. Grab the bar with a firm underhand grip and lift it up to your upper thighs, as shown. Maintain an upright posture. Brace your core.

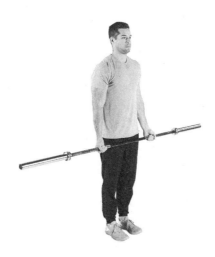

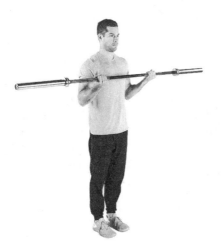

Action: Keeping your upper arms and elbows close to your sides, curl the bar up to your upper chest. Lower the bar to the starting position, moving through a full range of motion. This completes one rep.

CLOSE GRIP BENCH PRESS

Start: Lie down on your back on a bench. Grasp the barbell and position your hands fairly close together. Lift the bar and hold it directly above you with your arms extended.

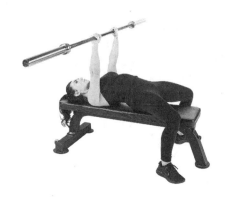

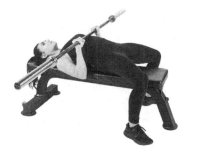

Action: Move the bar down slowly, keeping your elbows in, until you feel it on your chest. Pause for a second and return the bar to the starting position. This completes one rep.

Ball Crunch (see page 132)

Workout 2

Combat Stretch (see page 146)
Single Leg Toe Touch (see page 148)
Pelvic Tilts (see page 158)

BODYWEIGHT HIP THRUST

Start: Lie on your back on the floor or exercise mat with your knees bent. Extend your arms out to your sides.

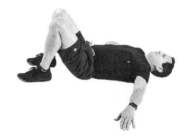

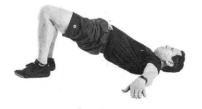

Action: Pressing through your heels, lift your hips off the floor, so that your hips form a straight line with your knees and shoulders. Squeeze your glutes at the top of the movement. Lower your torso back to the floor. Continue lifting and lowering for 1 minute.

BARBELL DEADLIFT

Start: Place the barbell on the floor in front of your feet and keep your legs close to the bar. Your feet should be about hip-width apart. Take a shoulder-width grip on the bar. Keep your back and arms straight.

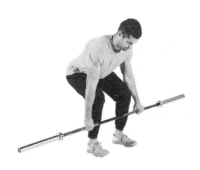

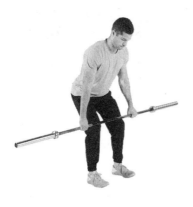

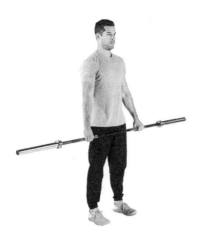

Action: Pull the bar up the front of your thighs, using the strength of your legs. At the top of the movement, squeeze your glutes, and pull your shoulders back.

To return the bar to the floor, push your bottom backward and lower the bar down the front of your legs, keeping your back straight. Place the barbell back on the floor. This completes one rep.

FARMER WALKS

Start: Grasp a dumbbell
in each hand. Stand
straight with good posture;
tighten your core and
shoulder blades. Squeeze
your glutes.

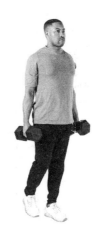

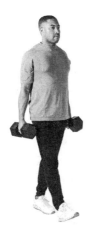

Action: Simply start
walking for a total of
20 steps.

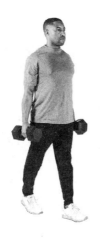

INCLINE DUMBBELL PRESS

Start: Set your bench at an incline, and grasp two dumbbells with an overhand grip. Bring the dumbbells to the sides of your body at chest level. Plant your feet firmly on the floor.

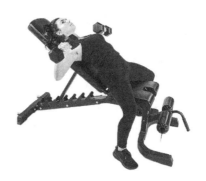

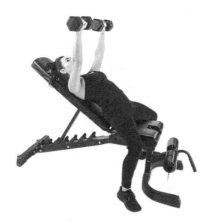

Action: Press the dumbbells straight up overhead, holding them directly over your chest and slightly touching each other with your palms facing forward. Slowly bend your elbows and lower both dumbbells in a slow, controlled fashion to the sides of your chest. This completes one rep.

Dumbbell Overhead Press (see page 152)

REAR DELT FLYS

Start: Lie facedown on a 45-degree angled exercise bench, as shown, balancing on your toes. Grasp a dumbbell in each hand. Maintain a slight bend in your elbows.

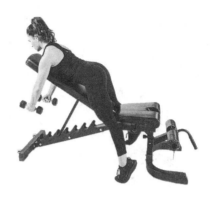

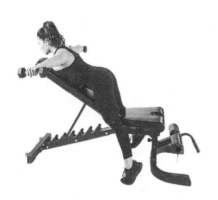

Action: Raise your arms up and out to your sides until your shoulder blades want to retract. Return the dumbbells to the starting position. This completes one rep.

Hammer Curls (see page 153)

DUMBBELL LYING TRICEPS EXTENSION

Start: Lie on your back on a flat exercise bench and grasp one dumbbell with both hands or grasp a dumbbell in each hand. Extend your arms upward, as shown, with the weight over your head.

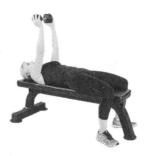

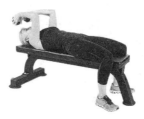

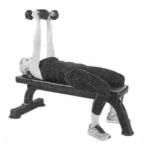

Action: Bend your arms at your elbows only, keeping your elbows fixed and pointing at your hips. Slowly lower the dumbbells down beside your head until they are about level with your ears.

Then, raise the dumbbells back to the starting position. This completes one rep. Be sure to move through a full range of motion.

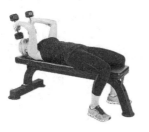

Band Chop (see page 123)

THE ROUTINE

In this routine, choose from one to three sets for all phases. This one is also phased by reps.

Exercises	Phase 1			Phase 2			Phase 3		
	Week 1	Week 2	Week 3	Week 4	Week 5	Week 6	Week 7	Week 8	Week 9
Workout 1 (Monday and optional Friday)									
90/90 Primer	1 minute	1 minute	1 minute	1 minute	1 minute	1 minute	1 minute	1 minute	1 minute
Combat Stretch	1 minute	1 minute	1 minute	1 minute	1 minute	1 minute	1 minute	1 minute	1 minute
Windmill	1 minute	1 minute	1 minute	1 minute	1 minute	1 minute	1 minute	1 minute	1 minute
Box/Bench Squats	▪1 to 3 sets ▪6 to 8 reps	▪1 to 3 sets ▪6 to 8 reps	▪1 to 3 sets ▪6 to 8 reps	▪1 to 3 sets ▪10 to 12 reps	▪1 to 3 sets ▪10 to 12 reps	▪1 to 3 sets ▪10 to 12 reps	▪1 to 3 sets ▪15 to 20 reps	▪1 to 3 sets ▪15 to 20 reps	▪1 to 3 sets ▪15 to 20 reps
Barbell Squats	▪1 to 3 sets ▪6 to 8 reps	▪1 to 3 sets ▪6 to 8 reps	▪1 to 3 sets ▪6 to 8 reps	▪1 to 3 sets ▪10 to 12 reps	▪1 to 3 sets ▪10 to 12 reps	▪1 to 3 sets ▪10 to 12 reps	▪1 to 3 sets ▪15 to 20 reps	▪1 to 3 sets ▪15 to 20 reps	▪1 to 3 sets ▪15 to 20 reps
Barbell Bench Press	▪1 to 3 sets ▪6 to 8 reps	▪1 to 3 sets ▪6 to 8 reps	▪1 to 3 sets ▪6 to 8 reps	▪1 to 3 sets ▪10 to 12 reps	▪1 to 3 sets ▪10 to 12 reps	▪1 to 3 sets ▪10 to 12 reps	▪1 to 3 sets ▪15 to 20 reps	▪1 to 3 sets ▪15 to 20 reps	▪1 to 3 sets ▪15 to 20 reps
Barbell Row	▪1 to 3 sets ▪6 to 8 reps	▪1 to 3 sets ▪6 to 8 reps	▪ 1 to 3 sets ▪6 to 8 reps	▪1 to 3 sets ▪10 to 12 reps	▪1 to 3 sets ▪10 to 12 reps	▪1 to 3 sets ▪10 to 12 reps	▪1 to 3 sets ▪15 to 20 reps	▪1 to 3 sets ▪15 to 20 reps	▪1 to 3 sets ▪15 to 20 reps
Barbell Overhead Press	▪1 to 3 sets ▪6 to 8 reps	▪1 to 3 sets ▪6 to 8 reps	▪1 to 3 sets ▪6 to 8 reps	▪1 to 3 sets ▪10 to 12 reps	▪1 to 3 sets ▪10 to 12 reps	▪1 to 3 sets ▪10 to 12 reps	▪1 to 3 sets ▪15 to 20 reps	▪1 to 3 sets ▪15 to 20 reps	▪1 to 3 sets ▪15 to 20 reps
Barbell Curls	▪1 to 3 sets ▪ 6 to 8 reps	▪1 to 3 sets ▪6 to 8 reps	▪1 to 3 sets ▪6 to 8 reps	▪1 to 3 sets ▪10 to 12 reps	▪1 to 3 sets ▪10 to 12 reps	▪1 to 3 sets ▪10 to 12 reps	▪1 to 3 sets ▪15 to 20 reps	▪1 to 3 sets ▪15 to 20 reps	▪1 to 3 sets ▪15 to 20 reps

continues

continued

Exercises	Phase 1			Phase 2			Phase 3		
	Week 1	Week 2	Week 3	Week 4	Week 5	Week 6	Week 7	Week 8	Week 9
Close Grip Bench Press	▪1 to 3 sets ▪6 to 8 reps	▪1 to 3 sets ▪6 to 8 reps	▪1 to 3 sets ▪6 to 8 reps	▪1 to 3 sets ▪10 to 12 reps	▪1 to 3 sets ▪10 to 12 reps	▪1 to 3 sets ▪10 to 12 reps	▪1 to 3 sets ▪15 to 20 reps	▪1 to 3 sets ▪15 to 20 reps	▪1 to 3 sets ▪15 to 20 reps
Ball Crunch	▪1 to 3 sets ▪6 to 8 reps	▪1 to 3 sets ▪6 to 8 reps	▪1 to 3 sets ▪6 to 8 reps	▪1 to 3 sets ▪10 to 12 reps	▪1 to 3 sets ▪10 to 12 reps	▪1 to 3 sets ▪10 to 12 reps	▪1 to 3 sets ▪15 to 20 reps	▪1 to 3 sets ▪15 to 20 reps	▪1 to 3 sets ▪15 to 20 reps
Workout 2 (Wednesday)									
Combat Stretch	1 minute	1 minute	1 minute	1 minute	1 minute	1 minute	1 minute	1 minute	1 minute
Single Leg Toe Touch	▪1 to 3 sets ▪6 to 8 reps	▪1 to 3 sets ▪6 to 8 reps	▪1 to 3 sets ▪6 to 8 reps	▪1 to 3 sets ▪10 to 12 reps	▪1 to 3 sets ▪10 to 12 reps	▪1 to 3 sets ▪10 to 12 reps	▪1 to 3 sets ▪15 to 20 reps	▪1 to 3 sets ▪15 to 20 reps	▪1 to 3 sets ▪15 to 20 reps
Pelvic Tilts	1 minute	1 minute	1 minute	1 minute	1 minute	1 minute	1 minute	1 minute	1 minute
Bodyweight Hip Thrust	1 minute	1 minute	1 minute	1 minute	1 minute	1 minute	1 minute	1 minute	1 minute
Barbell Deadlift	▪1 to 3 sets ▪6 to 8 reps	▪1 to 3 sets ▪6 to 8 reps	▪1 to 3 sets ▪6 to 8 reps	▪1 to 3 sets ▪10 to 12 reps	▪1 to 3 sets ▪10 to 12 reps	▪1 to 3 sets ▪10 to 12 reps	▪1 to 3 sets ▪15 to 20 reps	▪1 to 3 sets ▪15 to 20 reps	▪1 to 3 sets ▪15 to 20 reps
Farmer Walks	▪1 to 3 sets ▪20 steps	▪1 to 3 sets ▪20 steps	▪1 to 3 sets ▪20 steps	▪1 to 3 sets ▪20 steps	▪1 to 3 sets ▪20 steps	▪1 to 3 sets ▪20 steps	▪1 to 3 sets ▪20 steps	▪1 to 3 sets ▪20 steps	▪1 to 3 sets ▪20 steps
Incline Dumbbell Press	▪1 to 3 sets ▪6 to 8 reps	▪1 to 3 sets ▪6 to 8 reps	▪1 to 3 sets ▪6 to 8 reps	▪1 to 3 sets ▪10 to 12 reps	▪1 to 3 sets ▪10 to 12 reps	▪1 to 3 sets ▪10 to 12 reps	▪1 to 3 sets ▪15 to 20 reps	▪1 to 3 sets ▪15 to 20 reps	▪1 to 3 sets ▪15 to 20 reps
Dumbbell Overhead Press	▪1 to 3 sets ▪6 to 8 reps	▪1 to 3 sets ▪6 to 8 reps	▪1 to 3 sets ▪6 to 8 reps	▪1 to 3 sets ▪10 to 12 reps	▪1 to 3 sets ▪10 to 12 reps	▪1 to 3 sets ▪10 to 12 reps	▪1 to 3 sets ▪15 to 20 reps	▪1 to 3 sets ▪15 to 20 reps	▪1 to 3 sets ▪15 to 20 reps
Rear Delt Flys	▪1 to 3 sets ▪6 to 8 reps	▪1 to 3 sets ▪6 to 8 reps	▪1 to 3 sets ▪6 to 8 reps	▪1 to 3 sets ▪10 to 12 reps	▪1 to 3 sets ▪10 to 12 reps	▪1 to 3 sets ▪10 to 12 reps	▪1 to 3 sets ▪15 to 20 reps	▪1 to 3 sets ▪15 to 20 reps	▪1 to 3 sets ▪15 to 20 reps

continues

continued

Exercises	Phase 1			Phase 2			Phase 3		
	Week 1	Week 2	Week 3	Week 4	Week 5	Week 6	Week 7	Week 8	Week 9
Hammer Curls	▪1 to 3 sets ▪6 to 8 reps	▪1 to 3 sets ▪6 to 8 reps	▪1 to 3 sets ▪6 to 8 reps	▪1 to 3 sets ▪10 to 12 reps	▪1 to 3 sets ▪10 to 12 reps	▪1 to 3 sets ▪10 to 12 reps	▪1 to 3 sets ▪15 to 20 reps	▪1 to 3 sets ▪15 to 20 reps	▪1 to 3 sets ▪15 to 20 reps
Dumbbell Lying Triceps Extension	▪1 to 3 sets ▪6 to 8 reps	▪1 to 3 sets ▪6 to 8 reps	▪1 to 3 sets ▪6 to 8 reps	▪1 to 3 sets ▪10 to 12 reps	▪1 to 3 sets ▪10 to 12 reps	▪1 to 3 sets ▪10 to 12 reps	▪1 to 3 sets ▪15 to 20 reps	▪1 to 3 sets ▪15 to 20 reps	▪1 to 3 sets ▪15 to 20 reps
Band Chop	▪1 to 3 sets ▪6 to 8 reps	▪1 to 3 sets ▪6 to 8 reps	▪1 to 3 sets ▪6 to 8 reps	▪1 to 3 sets ▪10 to 12 reps	▪1 to 3 sets ▪10 to 12 reps	▪1 to 3 sets ▪10 to 12 reps	▪1 to 3 sets ▪15 to 20 reps	▪1 to 3 sets ▪15 to 20 reps	▪1 to 3 sets ▪15 to 20 reps

HIIT IT!

As I mentioned earlier, the form of aerobic exercise I recommend is HIIT (high-intensity interval training), as long as it is appropriate for your fitness level. Start slowly if you are a beginner because HIIT is intense.

The most effective way to do it, however, is to combine it with resistance training. It burns just as many calories as when you do HIIT on a cardio machine, with the added benefits of muscle development, strength gain, and body sculpting.

One challenge, though, is that resistance training requires much more planning. You must pick the right exercises and put them in the right order to make them more effective than sprinting on a cardio machine. Haphazardly organized resistance training exercises can increase your risk of injury *and* you lose most of the benefits.

Not to worry. Here is a well-programmed HIIT routine with an excellent track record of success with my clients. This workout is based on bodyweight only exercise, meaning you don't even need access to a gym or any workout equipment at all.

Do the following workout three days a week for maximum fat-burning and metabolism-boosting effects.

- Bodyweight Squats: 45 seconds (page 117)
- Rest: 15 seconds
- Push-Ups: 25 seconds (page 118)
- Rest: 15 seconds
- Prone Cobra Primer: 30 seconds (page 116)
- Rest: 15 seconds
- Plank: 25 seconds (page 165)
- Rest: 15 seconds
- Stationary Lunge: 20 seconds (page 127)
- Rest until your heart rate comes back down.
- Repeat until you have worked out for 15 minutes.

The tempo for these exercises should be controlled and moderate. Not superfast, but also not very slow. Just a continuous moderate pace. Make sure to take the prescribed rest periods *even if* you feel you don't need them. If you just go from exercise to exercise with no rest, you will essentially be doing steady state cardio and will miss out on the benefits of HIIT. After performing a round, rest for as long as it takes for your heart rate to come down. As you get fitter, you will need less rest at the end of each round. Never rest for less than forty-five seconds. Do as many rounds as you can for fifteen minutes and take longer breaks and rest periods, if necessary.

PART 3

INTUITIVE NUTRITION FOR PERMANENT FAT LOSS

10

THE ONLY DIET STRATEGY
YOU'LL EVER NEED

Y ou know it, and I know it: It's hard to begin a diet, much less stay on one! You feel deprived from the get-go, you're nagged by cravings, and you're at war with what to eat and what not to eat. Eventually, out of sheer frustration, you ditch that diet, and back come the pounds.

I've consistently seen this pattern in clients who dieted too hard and restricted too much food too quickly. Like clockwork, they'd lose weight, only to find it right back on their body shortly afterward.

As with so many people, my clients were reeled in by diet books that promised to get them lean and healthy in the fastest or best way possible. Some of these diets were low carb and high fat, whereas others were low fat and high carb. Some were high in animal foods (or even exclusively, such as the carnivore diet), whereas others were plant-based or vegan.

There are diets that have you drinking celery juice and others that have you knocking back cabbage juice. There are diets based on how people in Mediterranean regions eat, and others based on how people in Okinawa or Seventh-Day Adventists in Loma Linda, California, eat. All of them are different, but all of them promise the same thing: fast and easy results.

Here's the problem: Most of these diets are simply not sustainable. They do not give you enough satisfaction, satiety, or nourishment. They limit food variety and food quantity, which can bring on cravings and hunger pangs. They don't teach or help you to make smarter food choices, and they can be the very cause of an unhealthy relationship with food. They focus on the "how" you gain or lose weight, but they ignore the "why."

Nor are they individualized to your unique physiology. I have yet to see a diet that works over the long term, or is tailored to a person's preferences or lifestyle. Fortunately, there is a better way. It is called intuitive eating. Customized to how you live, it is the only way to achieve sustainable results.

WHAT IS INTUITIVE EATING?

The best way to describe intuitive eating is to look at how intuitive eaters live their lives:

They reject rigid food rules. They discover that healthy foods, such as lean proteins, vegetables, fruits, and natural carbohydrates, taste good and make their body feel better. They reject junk food binges.

They honor their hunger signals. Intuitive eaters are very skilled at distinguishing between physical hunger and emotional hunger due to loneliness, boredom, anger, and so forth—and eat accordingly. They also stop eating when they're satisfied, or close to it. They listen to their body's own cues to decide what, when, and how much to eat.

They are at peace with food. They don't feel guilty if they eat something that's off most diets. Nor do they beat themselves up over their choices. They simply enjoy the indulgence and move on.

They love and respect their body, knowing that it is designed to last a lifetime when given the proper resources, such as good nutrition and physical activity. They still want to improve their shape and performance, while appreciating all the wonderful things their body can do for them.

They embrace exercise and know that it brings their body joy, lifts their moods, and contributes to long-term health.

They understand the value of nutrition—how it supports strength, fitness, and health—and they naturally gravitate toward a more nutritionally balanced way of eating.

They can be carnivores, vegans, vegetarians of all kinds, whole food, plant-based, Paleo—whatever meets nutritional requirements and personal preference. They do not sacrifice nutritional health on the altar of their chosen plan.

They recognize how good intuitive eating feels. It is not a diet; it is just living your life in a way that feels natural but is also healthy and sustainable. Intuitive eating is about doing what feels natural and not about forcing yourself into a round-hole, square-peg way of dieting.

THE STAGES OF INTUITIVE EATING

How can you become an intuitive eater? As with anything new, it takes practice, commitment, and perseverance to get to a place where you eat intuitively. It doesn't happen overnight. In fact, there are four stages of intuitive eating.

The first stage is *unconscious incompetence*. In this stage, you haven't learned about how to eat for your overall health, or even what to eat. Put another way, you simply don't know what you don't know. If you're brand-new to resistance training and nutrition, you're probably at this stage. Fortunately, though, you can move out of this stage pretty quickly, especially if you're committed to changing your food and exercise habits.

The second stage is *conscious incompetence*. Here, you're learning the basics, such as how many macronutrients, or "macros" (protein, carbohydrates, and fats), your body needs for optimum muscular development and fat loss. You have become aware of what you don't know. Such tools as food trackers, into which you enter your calories and grams of macros so as to accomplish your goals, help.

The third stage is *conscious competence*. You're becoming mindful of the food you eat, its amount, and how it affects you, physically and psychologically. Through regular food tracking, you've begun to master your calories and macros and are getting a handle on exactly what to eat to get lean and physically healthy. You know what to do for better health, but you have to consciously do it. It is not automatic.

You don't have to stay here forever, however. It can become pathological and stressful to always count calories and macros, day in and day out. No one wants to live in a space where everything needs to be tracked forever.

The final stage is *unconscious competence*—the stage at which intuitive eating is in its full glory. No longer do you have to consciously think about what you know. Nor do you have to track your food anymore. You know when you're full and when to stop eating. You're intuitively making nutritious food choices, practically without thinking about them. You know how to fuel yourself to feel great and stay energized. You've arrived, and you're in the flow of intuitive eating.

Think of these four stages as similar to learning how to ride a bicycle. When you first got on a bike, you started in the first stage, knowing nothing about how to master it. At first, you probably fell over sideways on the bike a few times and scraped your knees. But in the second stage, once you got back on the bike, you wobbled a bit but without falling.

Through practice, you progressed to the third stage in which you had to really focus on your balance and your feet, legs, and hands to be able to ride your bike. Eventually, with enough practice, riding your bike became automatic as you moved into the fourth stage.

With intuitive eating, you eat in a healthy manner because *you want to*! How fabulous would that be? Making proper food choices is no longer a struggle, rather, a boost to the health of your mind and body. You trust yourself and your body again. You gain food freedom and flexibility because no longer is food your master. You are the master over food.

HOW TO GET STARTED WITH INTUITIVE EATING

Stay Consistent with Resistance Training

Intuitive eating is intimately related to physical activity. In fact, there is another huge benefit of resistance training that I haven't shared with you yet: starting regular workouts will inspire you to eat more healthfully—and intuitively. It's true! After you add physical activity to your life, the consequence is not only a great body but also significant, almost automatic changes in the way you eat.

This isn't just my observation from working with clients. It has been proven to be a fact from a 2019 study conducted at Stanford University. Researchers found that 2,000 of 2,500 college students who started exercising began to *naturally* eat more nutritious foods, such as fruits, vegetables, lean meats, fish and nuts, and fewer fried foods, sodas, and snack foods. It was as if they were on automatic pilot when it came to selecting nutritious foods. Plus, the more—and more vigorously—people exercised, the more their diet tended to improve.

Exercise, therefore, is the single best place to begin if you want to eat intuitively. It helps you effortlessly eliminate all the white-knuckling and teeth-gritting it takes to avoid certain foods and stick to a diet (that is bound to fail). You will find yourself making healthier food choices, naturally.

Eat with Awareness

It is very important to listen to your body when deciding how much and what to eat. So, as mealtime approaches, ask yourself whether you are truly hungry. Many times, thirst can masquerade as hunger. In other situations, we eat because we are sad, depressed, anxious, bored, lonely, or even happy. This is "emotional hunger." It's better to eat when you're physically hungry.

When planning meals, take a minute to ask yourself what food will truly nourish you from a physical, mental, and emotional perspective. Do this honestly, and you'll find that you choose foods that best serve your physical self. Less often, you may find that you make food choices that serve your mental and emotional self. For example, you may be visiting friends you haven't seen for a while, and a few glasses of wine and some nostalgic comfort foods are perfect for friendship bonding.

Find a place to sit down that is quiet and not distracting, so that you are aware of the food you are eating. Awareness helps prevent bingeing or eating too fast. Appreciate the food's taste, texture, and smell. Liquefy your food with chewing. Consciously enjoy the taste of your food from the moment it goes into your mouth until you swallow it. You should not need any fluids while eating; in fact, avoid beverages while eating. They can dilute digestive enzymes and make you too full prior to getting adequate nutrition. Take your time.

Practicing awareness during a meal is about slowing down, being fully mindful of what is happening within and around you at the moment. A growing body of science suggests that eating with awareness can help with weight problems, compulsive overeating, and eating disorders—plus, motivate us to make more healthful food choices.

Here are some additional strategies that can build the habit of awareness into your mealtimes:

- Stop multitasking at meals. In other words, turn off the TV or your phone, put away that novel or newspaper, and simply focus on eating your meal.
- Eat only at your dining table—no eating at your desk, in your car, or in bed. This ties eating with a specially designated spot.
- Eat slowly and chew your food well. Not only will you get greater satisfaction from less food, but you also give your body time to tell you that you are full. Avoid drinking while eating. It is not only better for digestion but prevents washing down big pieces of food quickly.
- Focus on each mouthful—its taste, texture, and smell.
- Eat with your nondominant hand. Or eat with chopsticks, if you don't ordinarily use them. This slows down your eating quite a bit.
- Put your fork or spoon down between bites—which also slows you down and helps prevent overeating.

You may find that, at times, you will resist being totally present and aware around food choices and eating. This is because being aware forces us to acknowledge our choices. This is tough but worth it. Always fight the urge to eat mindlessly or without awareness.

After your meal, pass no judgment on yourself. Simply observe and take note of how you felt before, during, and after you have a meal. For example, ask yourself:

- How hungry were you before your meal? (on a scale from 1 to 10, with 10 being very hungry)
- How hungry are you after the meal? (same scale)
- Are you satisfied or stuffed?
- Are you stressed, annoyed, anxious, happy, or sad?
- Did you eat quickly or slowly?
- Are you sleepy or energized?

You might be tempted to criticize your decisions, and say, "Next time, I won't eat this or that" or "Next time, I will eat less or eat more." Don't fall into this trap. It's a judgment game that only stifles your ability to read your body. Guilt, regret, and judgment are anti-awareness. So are self-hate, self-disgust, or self-disappointment. These emotions make you feel bad about yourself. Although they may drive you to eat "healthy" in the short term, they lead to eating patterns that promote weight fluctuations, cravings, and a poor relationship with food. You always want to eat from a place of self-care and self-love. Eating, after all, is an act of nourishment.

Connect Food to Physical Feelings

Keep a simple journal of how food makes you feel—both the positive and negative signals, but place special emphasis on the positive. Connecting certain foods, macro counts, and calories to positive body signals will change how you perceive specific foods. For example, you may not be particularly fond of the taste of vegetables, but if you consciously connect a sense of well-being, good energy, and normal digestion to each time you eat a serving of veggies, then you'll likely start to perceive the taste of vegetables as more desirable. In my case, when my digestion is off, I intuitively crave foods that help with my digestion. (See the following list of positive signals to look for.)

You may really enjoy a particular dish because it has some sort of meaning to you. Perhaps your mom made it, and it was your favorite food as a kid. We enjoy foods for more than just the taste. Building a good awareness around the positives regarding food, aside from just flavor, creates a healthy desire for foods.

On the flip side, you may find that carbs from fruit give you gas or cause bloating. For some people, proteins from dairy are intolerable (I am one of these people), and fats from animal products might cause you to feel lethargic.

This feedback is very important because, over time, it leads you to a place where you eat what is truly good for you because you want to. Eating intuitively gives you a new sense of enjoyment and satisfaction in your life, and it's worth doing whatever it takes to get to a healthy place in your relationship with your body.

Avoid Heavily Processed Foods

If I could give only one piece of advice to anyone in regard to nutrition and intuitive eating, it would be this: avoid heavily processed foods. This is my only hard-and-fast rule around intuitive eating.

Heavily processed foods are typically foods found in boxes or wrappers, and they usually have a long shelf life, thanks to preservatives and additives. Think: chips, cookies, muffins, cereal, bread products, and so forth. While learning to eat intuitively, you are probably better off avoiding these foods.

Earlier I mentioned that a diet high in heavily processed foods naturally led people to eat 500 more calories per day, according to one study. Well, that same study showed that people also ate much *faster* when they consumed heavily processed foods, averaging about 17 more calories per minute. Heavily processed foods *make* us eat more food and eat it faster!

What exactly is going on? Aside from the fact that they are usually not very healthy, heavily processed foods are radically engineered to hijack your body's natural systems of satiety. This engineering

POSITIVE SIGNALS THAT YOUR NUTRITION IS ON THE RIGHT TRACK

- Calm, even, and consistent energy
- Moderately elevated mood
- Sound, restful sleep
- Regular, fully formed bowel movements
- Clear, supple skin
- Bright eyes
- Preference for healthy foods
- Strong, healthy, and shiny hair
- Strong, fast-growing nails
- Strong immune system (you rarely get sick)
- Tolerance to contrasts in temperature
- Neutral body and breath odor
- Easy fat loss
- Easy muscle and strength development
- Fast recovery after workouts
- Healthy and fulfilling libido
- Stress resilience
- Sharp mind and thinking

includes everything that makes food truly enjoyable, including its taste, the mouthfeel, its smell, the color and visual appeal, the sound the food makes when you bite into it, the food's packaging, and much more. Lots of money is plowed into researching and figuring out how to make foods irresistible. In other words, these foods are designed to make you want to overeat.

Reducing or eliminating heavily processed foods is challenging, especially if your current diet is high in these foods. Your brain is so hooked on their engineered palatability, and has adapted to their pleasure signals, that whole natural foods may taste boring and bland to you.

But once you stay away from these foods for long enough (usually a month or so), and replace them with nutritious, whole, natural foods, you will find that your brain and body will adapt so that these foods begin to taste better and you will start to slowly lose your desire for processed foods.

What's more, after you eat natural foods, your body will usually tell you when it's had enough rather than have this signal be short-circuited by heavily processed foods.

Best of all: If you restrict or eliminate heavily processed foods, including liquid calories in the form of commercial juices, sodas, and other calorie- and sugar-containing beverages, you begin automatically shedding body fat as your natural systems of appetite and satiety normalize. Plus, you'll feel better and enjoy even better health. Eating a whole foods diet of more vegetables, fruits, nuts and seeds, and unprocessed meats helps build your immune system and guard against disease.

Learn to Make Peace with Food

Sometimes you may *want* to eat a specific food based on the situation, such as a family gathering or celebration with those you love. This is fine, and indeed a good idea at times, because it can nurture your mental health.

For example, let's say it's Christmas and you are visiting with family that you haven't seen in a while. Your aunt brings her famous apple pie and your dad wants to have a glass of wine with you. In that instance, it is very healthy for your mental and emotional health to foster relationships with your aunt and dad over those foods. Although that wine and apple pie might not be physiologically healthy, it was healthy overall. Intuitive eating is the ability to make these decisions with minimal thought and not feel guilty about it.

Also, you may choose to not eat that pie or drink that wine. But as I discussed in an earlier chapter, make your choices based on "I don't want that food at this time" rather than "I can't eat that food." There's a difference.

"I don't" is experienced as a choice, so it feels empowering and is an affirmation of your determination. "I can't" isn't a choice; it's a restriction you're imposing on yourself—the exact type of rule we are trying to get away from by being intuitive eaters. Saying "I can't" to food undermines your personal power.

Understand How Food Supports Muscle Development and Fat Burning

Part of the learning process on the way to becoming an intuitive eater has to do with understanding how food helps create muscle and burn fat. The most common reasons that people have trouble developing muscle and/or burning fat boil down to two main factors: They eat too many calories, or too little if the goal is to develop muscle, and they do not consume optimal levels of the three macros.

If you go on a crash diet, for example, and slash your calorie intake, your body doesn't burn only fat for energy, it also reduces its muscle mass, thus slowing the metabolism.

If you're new to resistance training, and your body has fat stores it can rely on for energy, then resistance training will help you lose that fat and gain muscle at the same time. On the other hand, if your physique is lean and you already have some muscle mass but want to develop more, you would have to increase your calorie intake so that you don't lose muscle in the process. You'll learn in the next chapter how to plan your diet around these principles.

Make Food Choices out of Self-Love

Intuitive eaters make food choices based on how much they truly care about themselves and respect their body. They know that nutritious food makes them feel better, it supplies nutrients that support muscle development and fat loss, and it fuels their body with vital substances that extend the quality and potentially the quantity of life (longevity). They value and enjoy food for the flavor and healthy nourishment it brings to their life.

In contrast, if someone is filled with self-hate, his or her food choices will reflect this loathing. Ill health will be the result.

Self-love and self-respect toward your body take time to develop. This is especially true if you've been losing weight and putting it back on over the years. Start by giving yourself credit for trying.

Intuitive eating involves your attitude as well as your menu. Write down in your journal all the qualities you appreciate about your body and what it does for you. Concentrate on your positive attributes rather than dwell on your thick waistline.

Think: long term, not quick fix. Work toward changes you can permanently sustain. Keep in mind that the choices you make today can help you live longer and lower your risk for diabetes, heart disease, and other serious conditions.

Implement Intuitive Eating Days

After you feel comfortable giving yourself calories and macro targets, plan some "intuitive days." These are days during which you track your food, but you don't consciously aim for any targets. I look at these days as practice days. You are learning to read your body's signals. Eat when you are hungry, for example, and don't eat when you are not. Choose foods that your body is telling you to choose.

As you learn to read your body's signals, intuitive days will at first seem like "off days." That's okay. Don't judge them, and don't judge your decisions. This is all practice.

Gradually increase your intuitive days each week until all are intuitive days. After transitioning to intuitively eating every day, you may find yourself in a situation in which you have to resume food tracking. Just keep in mind that intuitive eating is a skill and takes time to master. Progress is not linear, and there is no end goal.

Go Slowly

If you want to really stay in shape and enjoy great health, your best approach is to proceed with slow and steady changes, not with dramatic shifts. The key here is in understanding that your pace will be unique to you. Look at your diet and find something you can change that will challenge you but also be something you know you can stick to in the long term. It may be a small change (such as eating an extra serving of veggies or cutting out sugar), but odds are higher that it will be a permanent change. Once a dietary improvement has become a natural part of your eating behavior, add in another small change, and so on. Before you know it, you will have achieved permanent success.

Becoming an intuitive eater can take a long time, so be patient. In my experience, the process can take between six months to a year. You are erasing old habits and building new ones. You are developing a good relationship with your body and with food. Along the way, you are producing healthy results, step-by-step. Once you get to the place of intuitive eating, the results are permanent and healthy.

Stay the course. Eventually eating healthy and maintaining a heathy body will become a stress-free natural process, and you will enjoy your newfound freedom and flexibility.

RAW FITNESS TRUTH #7

YOU CAN GET FAT ON A KETO DIET.

Although the ketogenic diet may seem new or cutting edge, it's actually an old medical diet. It was first used by doctors in the early twentieth century to control seizures in epileptic patients. This medically based ketogenic diet consisted of 80 percent fat, as few carbohydrates as possible, and a low to moderate amount of protein in the range of 15 to 20 percent of total calories. The incredibly high fat intake combined with the nonexistent carb intake forces the body to produce substances called ketones for energy since it can't produce sufficient glycogen (stored carbohydrate in

continues

continued

muscle tissue). It's these ketones that seem to control or mitigate some of the effects of certain neurological disorders.

Although keto has medical benefits for select people, it certainly isn't a magical diet for the masses. It doesn't give you fat-burning powers, and it doesn't promote performance improvements for most athletes. Like all diets, there is always an individual variance with how people may respond to keto. For some people, it may work for a while. For others, it won't.

That being said, I have seen too many people gain more body fat on a keto diet than I have seen who have lost weight and kept that weight off. The reason I see people gaining fat from a ketogenic diet relates to the psychology behind the diet—a factor we seldom consider. A ketogenic diet is extremely restrictive. Although all diets have a restrictive component, the ketogenic diet cuts out an entire macronutrient—carbohydrates.

Not eating any carbs forever severely limits your food choices and is overly rigid. Once someone feels that a diet is too restrictive to maintain (which happens to everyone I have ever known on a ketogenic diet), they reintroduce carbs back into their diet. And this is when all hell breaks loose.

It's not that carbs are so appetite-stimulating that former ketogenic dieters lose control (although some high-carb heavily processed food choices can stimulate appetite), it's that breaking free from restriction creates a binge environment. When coming off a ketogenic diet, you are very likely to consume a lot of carbs and exceed your calorie requirements. Every time I have had a client or known someone who went off keto, they gained a large amount of weight afterward. Every single time. Again, I want to stress, it's not the carbs but rather the overconsumption of calories that causes this. Thus, in my opinion, the ketogenic diet may actually be doing more harm than good.

11

MACROS TO ACCELERATE YOUR RESULTS

Whathat you eat and how you eat matters when it comes to resistance training. Great bodies are made not only in a gym setting but also in the kitchen. Proper nutrition supplies your body with the nutrients it needs to recover from your workouts, create new muscle, and even help you burn fat. So, what you eat is important, as is the amount of calories, but the type of food from which you obtain those calories is just as important.

THE POWER OF PROTEIN

Protein is an essential macronutrient made up of twenty building blocks called amino acids. Some amino acids can be made in the body and are not essential in your diet. Other amino acids are essential, meaning that your body cannot make them. You must obtain them from food.

Animal foods supply all the essential amino acids, whereas most plant proteins, such as legumes provide incomplete amino acids. You can, however, eat combinations of various plant proteins and obtain complete amino acids.

Protein provides the construction material for muscles and other body tissues, organs, hormones, and enzymes. It is necessary to repair, build, and maintain muscle. It also increases satiety, which is why it's so important to get enough protein when you're striving toward a fat-loss goal. In fact, protein provides the highest satiety of any macro nutrient. Diets high in protein tend to reduce food cravings.

Protein also has the highest thermic effect of food (TEF), compared to fat and carbohydrates. TEF refers to the amount of calories you burn just to digest the food you eat. Eating a larger percentage of protein daily means more of the calories you eat are burned off through TEF.

Unlike with fat and carbohydrates, the body does not store protein, and therefore has no tank to draw on when it needs new provisions—which is why you must eat protein with most meals, regardless of what diet you follow.

How Much Protein Do You Need?

Although the amount of protein you require depends on your weight, goals, and lifestyle, most people need 40 to 60 grams of protein a day, at the very minimum, although this amount is far from ideal, especially if you perform resistance training because it boosts your protein requirements. Higher-protein diets have been shown to be consistently better at promoting fat loss and muscle gain, speeding up the metabolism, and controlling hunger.

What is considered "high protein"? Roughly 0.5 to 1.0 gram of protein per pound of your body weight, if you are not obese and are at your average weight. Example: a 130-pound average to overweight (but not obese) woman would aim for roughly 78 to 130 grams of protein a day. (If you are more than 20 pounds overweight, use your lean body mass instead of total weight.)

If your goal is to burn fat, ramping up the protein in your diet can help you lose more fat and preserve more lean muscle, so you'd want to consume the upper-end amount of protein.

Protein and muscular development go hand in hand. If you're trying to develop muscle or hold on to the muscle you have while shedding fat, 0.8 grams per pound of body weight will give you all the benefits of protein.

Everyone is different, though. Experiment to find the right level of protein for your body. Start with the recommendations here, see how they make you feel, and try adjusting your protein level up or down to determine what amount works best for you.

What Are the Best Sources of Protein?

Good sources of protein include all animal meats, poultry, fish, eggs, and dairy as well as plant or vegan proteins, such as nuts, seeds, and legumes.

Animal Proteins

Bison

Cheeses

Chicken, white meat and
   dark meat

Cottage cheese

Duck

Eggs and egg whites

Greek yogurt

Lamb

Lean beef

Organ meats from
   well-sourced producers

Pork tenderloin

Salmon

Shellfish

Tuna

Turkey, white meat and
   dark meat

Venison

White fish, all varieties

Plant-Based Proteins

Legumes

Nuts

Seeds

Vegan cheeses

ESSENTIAL FAT

Throughout the '70s, '80s, and most of the '90s, dietary fat was accused of being a troublemaker, blamed for heart disease, cancer, and the growing obesity epidemic. Our own government guidelines told us to not eat too many fats, especially saturated fats, because they were "so unhealthy." This turned out to be mostly false. Studies show

GUIDE TO PROTEIN FOR SUPERIOR HEALTH AND PERFORMANCE

- Aim for organic, grass-fed beef versus nonorganic grain-fed beef. Grass-fed beef has a better nutrient and fatty acid profile, whereas grain-fed beef is believed by many authorities to trigger inflammation in the body.
- Purchase organic pasture-raised poultry and eggs. These are higher in nutrients and omega-3 fatty acids, which have many disease-fighting and fat-burning properties.
- Choose wild, well-sourced, or sustainably farmed fish over traditional commercially farmed fish, which has been shown to have higher levels of toxins and antibiotic residues.
- Eat smaller fish, such as sardines, more frequently, rather than larger fish, such as swordfish. The mercury content in smaller fish is lower. Mercury is a neurotoxin that can damage brain cells.
- If you can tolerate dairy foods, select unpasteurized, non-homogenized, organic, grass-fed milk. Pasteurization destroys enzymes and beneficial bacteria, and homogenization damages natural fats. Grain-fed cows produce milk that has a less favorable fatty acid profile.
- Avoid processed meat and meat products, such as sausages, salami, lunch meats, most bacon, and so forth. Processed meats have been linked to poor health and increased cancer risk in several studies.

that a higher-fat diet that comprises healthy fats, within the context of a diet that is low enough in calories to maintain a lean body, is typically perfectly healthy.

Fat is also an essential nutrient and must be consumed for simple survival. Fat helps our body function in terms of energy, nutrient absorption, cell growth, and organ protection. Adding fat to your diet also helps you feel full faster and longer. It makes food more tasty; this helps you eat fewer calories overall.

As for resistance training, fat plays a crucial role in hormone regulation—particularly that of testosterone and growth hormone—both of which are essential for developing lean muscle and strength. Oftentimes, my clients on very low fat diets had trouble building muscle.

People of a few cultures who consume a diet very high in fat are also very healthy. The Inuit people of northern Canada and Alaska and the Masai tribes of Kenya and northern Tanzania derive most of their calories from animal fats and display incredible health. Of course, these cultures' respective diet is also relatively low in calories for their caloric energy output.

How Much Fat Do You Need?

The daily essential fat requirement for most people is 40 to 70 grams, and this represents the minimum requirement. Some people feel great with more fat in their diet than what is deemed essential, whereas others do fine with less. If your carbs are very low, you can increase your calories from fat, without going overboard on your daily caloric intake.

What Are the Best Sources of Fat?

Generally, the healthiest sources of fat come from some plants and from well-raised, healthy animals and fish, although organic butter and full-fat dairy products are acceptable too. Grass-fed beef, pasture-raised eggs, and fish are excellent ways to obtain good fats.

Avocados	Fish oil
Avocado oil	Ghee (clarified butter)
Butter, organic	Lard and tallow (excellent
Coconut oil (can withstand	for cooking)
higher cooking	MCT oil
temperatures)	*Nuts

Olives	Seeds, such as black
Olive oil, extra-virgin	sesame, pumpkin, flax,
(avoid cooking with	and hemp seeds
olive oil to preserve its	
nutrition; use it cold)	

*Nuts are best consumed raw. Roasting nuts can make them inflammatory in some cases.

Avoid these unhealthy fats: trans fats found in processed foods; and highly refined polyunsaturated vegetable oils, such as peanut, corn, and soy oils. They are unstable at high temperatures and become inflammatory when used in cooking. They are also high in omega-6 fatty acids, which can be inflammatory. The typical American diet with all of its processed foods is overloaded with these fats.

CARBOHYDRATES—THE ENERGIZERS

A fuel source, carbohydrates are the sugars and starches found in fruits, vegetables, grains, dairy products, and many processed foods. Sugar is the simplest form of carbohydrate and is a natural constituent of some foods, most notably fruit. Types of sugar include fruit sugar (fructose), table sugar (sucrose), and milk sugar (lactose). These are classified as simple carbohydrates; they are broken down and digested very quickly in the body.

Starch is a complex carbohydrate, meaning it is made of multiple sugar units bonded together. Starch is found naturally in vegetables, grains, and legumes. These foods take a much longer time for you to break down and digest, primarily because they are good sources of fiber. Science suggests that dietary fiber helps reduce your risk of cardiovascular diseases, obesity, and type 2 diabetes.

Over the last several decades, carbohydrates have gotten some bad press. They have been blamed for the obesity epidemic and for most of our modern chronic health problems. The science on carbohydrates doesn't really back this up, however. Numerous examples of long-living societies and cultures consume a good deal of their calories from carbohydrates. Okinawans are among the longest-living people on earth, for example, and they eat a diet that is largely made up of carbohydrates.

How is this possible? Unlike our modern society, they don't eat many calories. Americans, however, overconsume calories and carbohydrates in the form of heavily processed foods, which lead to obesity, diabetes, and other health issues.

Of the three macros, carbohydrates are not essential, although they appear to be a prioritized source of energy. Carbs are easily converted into energy by the body and can be involved in fat formation.

That said, I do recommend that you manipulate your carbohydrate intake in certain cases. If you need to lose body fat, for example, scale back on your carb intake, along with following a lower-calorie diet. If you want to develop more muscle, or maintain the muscle you have, increase your carbs.

Carb manipulation goes back to the strategy of intuitive eating. As you cut back or increase your carbs, listen to your body. See how you feel and perform. Monitor whether you're losing weight or putting on lean muscle.

Some feel they perform best on a low-carb, high-fat diet. But typically, the more intense workouts you do, the better you will perform and feel with a diet that is higher in carbs.

If you are usually sedentary (I hope not!), then you may do better on a lower-carbohydrate diet. You may not need lots of fast energy so cutting carbs down could be an easy way to reduce calories.

"Bad" or poor-quality carbs are foods that are high in refined sugars and low in nutritional value. Examples include doughnuts, cookies, candy, and pastries. Even commercial fruit juices are high in refined sugar. Drinking these beverages is essentially drinking a glassful of sugar. Plus, juices are stripped of all the beneficial fiber from the whole fruit.

Now, I'm not saying you should stay away from sugar. We all know fruits are full of sugar. It's okay to eat fruit, but it's important to understand that sugar from fruits is not refined. Carbohydrate foods that are high in refined sugar will raise your blood sugar very quickly, resulting in a poor mood and cravings, and may be converted into body fat. Consequently, high-sugar, high processed–carb diets make getting lean virtually impossible.

"Good" sources of carbs tend to be complex carbohydrates that are full of nutrients that digest slowly in your body. Examples are fruits, vegetables, grains, and legumes. These types of carbs normally take a longer time to raise your body's glucose levels and help control hunger, especially when eaten with protein. A couple of caveats: Some people find grains to be inflammatory, which shows up as bloat and poor digestion, due to their gluten content. If you're avoiding gluten for this reason, watch out for foods labeled as "gluten free." They can be highly processed and full of additives and may be higher in calories than the foods they replace.

In fact, evidence shows that eating complex carbs can help you control your weight. In 2015, a study published in the *Annals of Internal Medicine* suggested that something as simple as eating 30 grams of fiber each day—from fruits, vegetables, and other high-fiber foods—can help you lose weight, lower your blood pressure, and improve your body's response to insulin (which helps prevent diabetes) just as effectively as a more complicated diet.

Fiber is a great weight-loss tool. It supports weight control by helping you feel full on fewer calories. To get this benefit, it's best to focus on eating carbohydrates that are unprocessed and rich in nutrients.

How Many Carbs Do You Need?

The Dietary Guidelines for Americans recommends that carbohydrates make up 45 to 65 percent of your total daily calories. So, if you get 2,000 calories a day, between 900 and 1,300 calories should be from carbohydrates. That translates to between 225 and 325 grams of carbs a day.

However, each person should have their own carbohydrate goal. Take me, for example, I do best on under 100 grams of carbs daily—which is "moderate." Most of my clients did best on a moderate-carb diet, especially if their goal was to lose body fat.

Carbs are found in many different types of foods:

*Low-Calorie, High-Fiber Carbs

Asparagus	Green beans
Bean sprouts	Green leafy vegetables
Bell peppers	Kale
Broccoli	Leeks
Brussels sprouts	Lettuce, all varieties
Cabbage, all varieties	Onions, all varieties
Cauliflower	Scallions
Celery	Spinach
Chard	Tomatoes
Chicory	Winter squash
Cucumbers	Yellow summer squash
Eggplant	Zucchini

A good rule of thumb is to eat a large serving of these vegetables at the beginning of your meal, especially if you tend to overconsume calories and would like to lose body fat. Seek variety too. The more colorful a plant food, the more nutrients it contains.

*Root Vegetables

Artichokes	Potatoes
Beets	Radishes
Carrots	Sweet potatoes
Celeriac	Turnips
Garlic	Yams
Parsnips	

These vegetables tend to be slightly higher in starch.

*Legumes

Beans (kidney, navy, pinto,   Lentils
   black, cannellini, and   Peas
   so forth)   Peanuts

*These foods are high in protein and make good protein substitutions in plant-based meals. They are also higher in starch.

*Grains

**Amaranth   Pastas (whole wheat,
Barley   **bean-based)
Breads (whole-grain, sprouted)   **Quinoa
**Buckwheat   **Rice
**Corn   **Sorghum
Millet   Wheat
**Oatmeal

*Many people have intolerances to grain-based foods, especially wheat and gluten-containing grains. These foods are very high in starch.
**These are gluten-free grains (though, if using oats, check their label to be sure they are GF-certified).

*Fruit

Apples   Grapes   Pineapple
Bananas   Kiwis   Plums
Blueberries   Lemons   **Raspberries
Cantaloupe   Limes   Strawberries
Cherries   Mangoes   Watermelon
Coconut   Peaches
Grapefruit   Pears

*Fruits can be easily overconsumed. For most people, one serving of fruit daily is ideal.
**Very high in fiber

PLANNING FOR FAT LOSS

Most people are interested in one, high-priority goal: lose body fat. Let's look at how to do that in the easiest way possible. Here are the steps:

Step #1: Build your metabolism first.

Before you even think about what to eat, or how much, concentrate on performing your regular resistance training program. It is what creates a faster metabolism—which is exactly what you require to move your body into fat-burning mode. When you do that, getting rid of body fat becomes so much easier because resistance training signals your body that more muscle is needed and more calories can be burned. So, starting now, concentrate on resistance training.

Step #2: Calculate your calories, along with your macros (especially protein).

For fat loss to occur, you must consume fewer calories than you burn, or to put it another way, you must be burning more calories than you consume.

Remember, calories are units of energy. They tell you how much energy is contained within food. Your body uses energy to function and to be alive. When you eat more calories than your body requires, those extra calories get packed away as body fat, increasing the size of your existing fat cells. When you burn fat, your body uses the energy stored in your fat cells to fuel your activity. This makes your fat cells shrink in size.

Download a food-tracking app, such as My Fitness Pal or Fat Secret, to help you. Track your intake for two weeks, but don't try to change anything yet. You're creating a baseline from which to make changes later. Simply take note of your calories and how many grams of fat, protein, and carbohydrate you typically consume.

At the end of two weeks, figure your average caloric intake for each week. Let's use the example of Vickie, who works out with weights two or three times a week, as I recommend in this book. Following this step, she calculated her average weekly calories to be 14,000, or 2,000 calories a day (her baseline).

Step #3: Reduce your daily caloric intake.

Once you have your weekly average—the baseline—reduce your calories by 200 to 600 a day. I recommend starting at the lower range to gauge how your body responds. So, in Vickie's case, she would reduce her calories by 200 a day, for a total of 1,800 daily. If you cut too many calories, you increase the risk of losing lean muscle tissue. Smaller changes are always easier to maintain—and sustain.

Follow this plan for three to four weeks. Monitor changes on your scale, in your mirror, and how your clothes fit. If you observe no changes or very few, reduce your calories by another 200 to 600 calories a day.

Step #4: Meet your protein goal.

Make sure you're hitting 0.5 up to 1.0 gram of protein per pound of bodyweight daily. If you weigh 160 pounds, for example, you'd want to eat 80 to 160 grams of protein daily.

If you have more than 20 pounds of weight to lose, figure your protein intake based on your ideal, or goal, weight. Say you want to weigh 130 pounds. Your protein intake would be 65 to 130 grams daily.

Step #5: Be intuitive about your fat and carbohydrate intake.

As for the mix of fat and carbs each day, figure out how much of these macros works for you while staying within your calorie range. Some people do well on a low-carb, higher-fat plan; others on a higher-carb, lower-fat diet. The key here is to listen to your body and monitor it. How is your satiety? Digestion? Weight loss? Mood? Energy levels? See what feels best and looks best, and go with it.

Some general guidelines: For a lower-carb diet, aim for fewer than 50 to 100 grams of carbs a day and eat the rest of your calories in healthy fats. However, don't eat fewer than 25 to 40 grams of fat a day.

I have seen this dietary approach work time and time again. Case in point: Angela, an on-and-off-again dieter who wanted to lose 15 pounds. She was running a couple of miles every day, lifting weights once a week, and doing Pilates classes regularly—all on 1,500 calories a day. But the body fat wasn't budging.

Angela told me, "I can't imagine eating any less or working out any more!"

I slowly increased her calories while she focused on strength building to get her metabolism to boost. Once I got her to be able to maintain her current weight on 2,300 calories a day (up from 1,500), we started cutting calories. I brought her down to 1,800 calories a day. The body fat started dropping like crazy and she was exercising far less.

BUILD STRENGTH AND DEVELOP MUSCLE

If your goal is to develop muscle, be consistent with resistance training and determine your baseline calories as described above.

Then, do not change your caloric intake for three weeks, but keep training to build your metabolism.

After three weeks, increase your calories by 50 to 150 per day. Follow this for two weeks.

Next, increase your calories again—by 50 to 150 a day. Repeat this process every two weeks.

Bump up your calories by increasing your intake from protein, fats, and carbohydrates. A calorie surplus is essential for muscle growth because your body now has excess calories to shuttle toward building more muscle.

If you notice a weight gain on your scale of a few pounds, this probably indicates muscle and/or water. However, if the gain is more than a few pounds, wait a few weeks before increasing your calories and try again.

Please monitor yourself:

- Men should aim to gain 0.5 to 1 pound per week.
- Women should aim to gain 0.25 to 0.5 pound or less per week.

On the other hand, if you're not gaining weight, check your strength levels. Are you getting stronger? In other words, can you do more reps, more weight, and so forth than last week? If so, you're still improving. And you're likely dropping body fat.

But if your strength is not improving and your weight on the scale is not going up, increase your caloric intake by 10 to 20 percent, and continue to monitor your progress.

SMASH FAT-LOSS PLATEAUS

The dreaded fat-loss plateau. You hop on the scale and nothing has changed for a while. What gives? You've been losing fat for weeks or even months and haven't strayed far from your diet or resistance training workouts. But you can't seem to get the scale to shift. It happens to all of us at one point or another. Stalled weight loss is incredibly frustrating, and incredibly common.

A plateau is another form of metabolic adaptation. Your body is getting smaller as you diet down, and burns fewer calories as it shrinks. Thus, your metabolism slows. This is inevitable.

Remember that: calories in < calories out = fat loss. Metabolic adaptation causes the "calories out" side of your equation to decrease. So, something in that equation needs to change for progress to resume. Follow these steps.

1. Identify whether you have really plateaued.

Before making any changes, be sure that you're really at a plateau.

When it comes to weight, fluctuations are normal. Your weight will be all over the place on a weekly basis and won't give you an accurate picture of your fat loss—which is why I suggest also taking body measurements of your chest, waist, hips, and thighs, using a simple cloth tape measure.

Don't obsess over what the scale says in a week's time. Look at your weight over a three- to four-week period. Your trend should be downward.

If your weight gets stuck, however, and your measurements haven't changed over that period, then you've likely plateaued, and it is time to make some changes.

2. Make sure you're measuring your food accurately.

Your food journal might look like:

1 steak: 460 calories
1 bowl of rice: 204 calories
Total calories: 664
But in reality, it should look like:
8 ounces rib eye: 658 calories
2 cups cooked rice: 340 calories
Total calories: 998

That's a difference of 334 calories, for just one meal. If you're aiming to eat 500 calories below maintenance levels, that essentially makes your fat loss efforts a wash.

To prevent this, tighten up on your measuring—at least until you can accurately eyeball your portions. The food items you should measure are:

- *Fat sources.* Avocados, nuts, cooking oils, and so forth. High-fat foods are also the most calorie dense and can easily add a sneaky couple hundred calories to your daily total.
- *Animal proteins.* Again, there's a huge caloric difference between "1 steak" and "8 ounces of rib eye."
- *Foods served in bowls.* One bowl of oatmeal or rice, for example, could add up to multiple servings, leaving hundreds of calories unaccounted for. Whip out your measuring cups!
- *Anything currently tracked as small, medium, or large.* For example, 1 medium banana, 1 large avocado. Lots of room for error here. Weigh them. A bit of measuring goes a long way toward your fat loss.

3. Undulate your calories.

Here is an effective hack to blast your body out of a plateau. It is called "undulating your calories." This simply means changing your calorie intake from day-to-day.

Here is an example: Thomas was working toward a 30-pound fat loss. His dietary strategy was to eat the same number of calories daily, with a 500-calorie deficit from his baseline. This worked for a while, then everything came to a grinding halt. No longer was he losing body fat.

I suggested that he undulate his calories through the week. Here is how he did it:

Monday	800-calorie deficit
Tuesday	0-calorie deficit
Wednesday	500-calorie deficit
Thursday	200-calorie surplus
Friday	1,000-calorie deficit
Saturday	700-calorie deficit
Sunday	700-calorie deficit

Like Thomas, if you are at a 500-calorie deficit most days, you have a 3,500-calorie deficit for the week. But by undulating your calories, your food intake varies from day-to-day. In my experience, undulating calories tends to reduce the effects of metabolic adaptation (the slowing down of your metabolism) and breaks you out of a plateau. It is much more like real life with some higher-calorie days and some lower-calorie days. It is also a stepping-stone to intuitive eating. Once you have become more in tune with your body, you may find that some days, you eat more food; some days, you eat less. As soon as Thomas started undulating his calories, his body fat started melting off again.

- *Add another resistance training day.* I would normally start most new clients' resistance training at 2 or 3 times per week. Adding another training day is a natural part of the progression of increasing training volume. Plus, most people are ready and excited to take on more.
- *Try LISS.* This stands for "low-intensity steady-state" cardio. Examples are walking, hiking, or riding your bike, in which you aim for a low level of exertion a continuous period of time. Along with increasing your resistance training session, LISS may help reverse your fat-loss plateau.

REVERSE DIETING: A REVOLUTIONARY STRATEGY

A dietary strategy I've often recommended is reverse dieting. It evolved from the aftermath of fitness and bikini competitions, in which competitors would diet down so stringently, with a severely calorie-restricted diet, and overdo cardio that afterward, their metabolism would virtually shut down. A return to normal eating after the competition would result in rapid, undesirable weight and fat gain. To prevent this, their coaches came up with the idea of reverse dieting.

Reverse dieting is an eating plan that involves gradually increasing your calories—usually by 50 to 100 calories a week—over a period of several weeks or months, to boost your metabolism and coax your body back into a fat-burning state. It is also an excellent maintenance strategy after you've lost weight. It helps you ease back into a normal, healthy eating pattern without gaining extra weight or fat.

Reverse dieting works, not only for competitors, but is also useful for anyone who has dieted stringently by slashing calories, has gone on habitual crash diets, or wants to maintain their weight loss. As a result of dieting—especially if a restrictive diet—your metabolism takes a beating. The body starts to adapt, slowing down your metabolism in an effort to conserve energy. This becomes problematic when you want to return to a normal diet and maintain your weight loss. When you try to eat normally again, your body piles on the pounds rather quickly.

To prevent this and rebuild your metabolism, follow these reverse dieting guidelines:

- Increase your calories by 50 to 100 calories per week above your baseline, which is the number of calories you've been consuming.
- Continue this caloric increase until you reach your target, prediet caloric intake.
- Be sure to keep your protein intake high, since protein is a metabolic booster.
- Prioritize consistent resistance training so as to develop muscle, which will then accelerate your metabolism. Muscle is metabolism.
- Limit cardio. Long sessions of steady-state cardio do little to create muscle, and they may even interfere with rebuilding your metabolism.
- Monitor your weight while reverse dieting. If you see a large jump in weight gain during any given week, scale back from the rate at which you're increasing your caloric intake.

Once you're satisfied with the amount of food you're eating, and your weight is stabilizing where you want it, stop adding calories, but continue with your resistance training program. Should you need to lose a few more pounds, your metabolism will be healthy and ready to burn fat.

Reverse dieting is an excellent postdiet solution that helps you transition to a more normal calorie intake, heals your metabolism, and helps keep your weight off once you've lost it.

For resistance training, you will likely get the best results by including all three macronutrients, chosen from the healthiest, most nutritious foods. Keep in mind: Protein is essential because its main job is to repair damaged cells and build new muscle tissue. Carbohydrates provide energy. Fat is also a source of energy and aids in hormone production. Next up is how to put this knowledge to work in creating intuitive meals.

RAW FITNESS TRUTH #8

EATING SMALL FREQUENT MEALS DOESN'T WORK.

I bet you've heard statements such as "If you don't eat frequently your body will go into starvation mode and it will store fat!" or "Eating small frequent meals speeds up your metabolism."

Well, guess what? This is a huge myth. I will explain more in a moment, but first a personal story. For more than twelve years, I ate every two to three hours religiously. But, mysteriously, I had a very tough time getting lean. Despite eating frequent meals, I was hungry all the time, and my energy was always low. I relied on such stimulants as coffee and caffeinated drinks to power through my day and my workouts.

Then, one day, I stumbled across an article discussing the benefits of short fasts—going for eight to fourteen hours without food. Normally, I would immediately discredit articles like this; however, it was backed by solid scientific research extolling the virtues of eating infrequently.

continues

continued

From an evolutionary standpoint, this idea made sense to me. Ancient humans ate infrequently. They did not have the pleasure nor the convenience of having food available six times a day. They ate very little until they killed something or came upon a cache of edible plants, then they feasted.

I dug deeper. I found that there are no studies supporting the "eat every two to three hours" dogma. None. Zero. Zilch. As a matter of fact, I discovered the opposite to be true. Study after study showed health benefits to eating less frequently: lower blood sugar, improved energy, and reduced inflammation.

I decided to test the short-term fasting concept on a population of one—me. I ate a very small breakfast and fasted until dinner. Expecting the worst, I thought my workout performance would suffer, and I'd die from hunger pangs.

Instead, the opposite happened. I felt more energy, and I was not hungry! After four weeks of eating in this fashion, I had become leaner than ever before. My performance in the gym improved, and I felt healthier. No longer did I have to lug food around with me to eat through the day. I realized that the whole multiple-meals rule was a big fallacy.

So, how did this fallacy come to be? Believe it or not, it all started with the breakfast cereal companies. Before the 1860s (when cold cereals were invented), most people did not eat breakfast. They'd wake up, barely eat anything or nothing at all, and go about their day. They ate their main meal early in the afternoon. Not very much food was consumed afterward.

The introduction of breakfast cereals changed all that. Food manufacturers began advertising this new product as the perfect food to be eaten in the morning. In short order, eating breakfast (and breakfast cereals) became a staple of the modern diet.

Much later on, protein powders and protein bars came on the scene. To push more of these products, manufacturers began promoting that eating frequently throughout the day would build more muscle and promote weight loss. These assertions were

continues

continued

based on shoddy science, but from a marketing standpoint, their claims paid off. A billion-dollar industry was created.

So, what about that science?

First off, eating small meals does not speed up your metabolism.

Remember, when you eat, you create a "thermic effect," which means your metabolism heats up and you begin to burn more calories. This fact is what the bar and powder manufacturers have used as scientific "proof" to verify their claims that eating more frequently boosts your metabolism.

But here is the real truth. The thermic effect derived from eating matches the number of calories being consumed. In other words, eat a small meal and get a small thermic effect. Eat a large meal and you get a large thermic effect. So, it doesn't really matter whether you eat your food in six meals or two; you get the same net thermic effect.

Second, I want to challenge the whole idea that your body goes into "starvation" mode if you don't eat every two to three hours. This belief is not supported by any science. In fact, starvation mode takes a lot longer than ten hours or even forty-eight hours. You can't "starve" yourself with responsible infrequent eating!

Third, blood sugar in healthy individuals has been shown to be lower overall with infrequent feedings. But if you eat too frequently throughout the day, your blood sugar tends to rise over the course of the day.

Fourth, research shows that short fasting periods induce a cellular cleanup process known as autophagy, whereby your cells get rid of waste faster and remain healthier. This, in turn, has been shown to increase life span and reduce total body inflammation and cancer risk.

Finally, let's take a look at the idea that your muscles will deteriorate if you don't feed them frequently. This is a joke and, in fact, some studies suggest the opposite effect. I've observed from working with clients that too frequent protein feedings actually desensitize the body to protein and lower its rate of protein

continues

continued

synthesis. Put another way, your body becomes less efficient at utilizing protein for muscle recovery and muscle adaptation. So, too many protein feedings may reduce how much protein your body uses for building muscle!

So, what is my advice? Eat less frequently—maybe two meals a day with a light breakfast. Most people do best with this approach. Or, if you are burning a ton of calories due to a strenuous lifestyle or workout regimen, try three meals.

I eat very little in the morning—maybe an apple—and I have a small protein shake after my workout at around two p.m. My main meal is in the evening, when I get home from work at around eight p.m.

So, try to eat fewer meals and see how you feel. You might be pleasantly surprised at how much more convenient it is and how much better your body responds. You may wish to continue to eat less frequently.

On the other hand, if you prefer to eat small bites throughout the day and you feel best doing so, then go for it as long as you are eating healthy and your calorie, fat, protein, and carbohydrate intake is appropriate for your body and your goals. Ultimately, eating frequency is largely up to personal preference.

12

INTUITIVE MEALS

Creating your ideal body has much to do with how much protein, fat, and carbohydrate you put on your plate—and the quality of those macros—along with consistent resistance training. However, if you turned to this chapter to get a "meal plan" that supports the workout programs in *The Resistance Training Revolution*, I'm about to disappoint you. But that disappointment won't last long after I explain the benefits of *not* having a meal plan.

Before I continue, let me define what I mean by "meal plan." I'm talking about a specific list of foods to eat at breakfast, lunch, dinner, and snacks. I'm *not* talking about planning out your meals in advance for bulk cooking and meal prep. That approach isn't specific to losing weight, or following a diet. It's just a smart way of planning meals for budget, time, and healthy eating.

Having someone like a trainer or a dietitian give you a meal plan makes sense, in theory. It tells you exactly what to eat, how much food to eat and when to eat it. If you just follow the plan, you'll get to your goals, right?

Wrong. When I trained people, I used to hand out meal plans. It seemed like a good idea—my clients got results—but no one could keep making progress or maintaining their results. This wasn't their fault though. The meal plans failed them; they didn't fail the meal plans.

The only time I've actually seen meal plans *work* is when they were followed by bodybuilders, bikini competitors, or elite athletes training for a specific contest or event. It wasn't about the food, it was about ensuring that their nutrient needs were met, or getting them super-lean for a contest. Even then, these meal plans weren't long term. They were designed with a specific time frame in mind. Afterward, the competitor usually ditched the meal plan. I remember one bikini contestant who packed on 30 pounds of fat after her competition!

For everyone else—and that's you—you don't need a meal plan. You are smarter and becoming more intuitive than any detailed plan of what you can and cannot eat. You have needs that change day by day, week by week, and sometimes even hour by hour.

5 REASONS MEAL PLANS DON'T WORK

1. Meal plans are too rigid and not intuitive.

Meal plans set forth a strict set of guidelines. They dictate what to eat, how much, and when. Sure, you might be able to follow the plan for a short period of time, but then life usually intervenes. Stress hits, and you ditch said meal plan for a relaxing night out with friends. Maybe you head out on a business trip. You can't stick to the prescribed meal plan, and you end up eating food that wasn't on the plan. Perhaps the weather turns unpredictably cold and you feel like something warming and comforting rather than the light salad specified by your meal plan. All of this is okay, and you shouldn't beat up on yourself for not following it. Meal plans just aren't designed to support real life.

2. Meal plans foster an all-or-nothing mentality.

Perhaps you follow your meal plan for a while, then you get bored with its rotating list of egg whites, spinach, brown rice, chicken, tuna, salad, and maybe a piece of fruit. Eventually, you never want to see another stupid piece of lettuce or baked chicken breast again. You start craving something sweet, such as ice cream or cake, so you detour from the meal plan and eat your sweets. Afterward, you say, "What the heck" and embark on an all-out binge.

You've lapsed into what psychologists call all-or-nothing thinking: "Well, I didn't stick to my meal plan, so I might as well eat everything in sight." This mind-set keeps you stuck and warps your relationship with food. You have trouble eating anything in moderation and are constantly yo-yoing from one extreme to another, flipping from restriction to binge eating. A meal plan only traps you further in this mind-set, without a clear path out.

3. Meal plans lack the ability to adapt to cultural preferences.

Very few diets out there take into consideration a person's heritage. This is a big problem. When people come to the United States from other countries, many don't abandon their traditional cuisine, but many others Americanize their eating habits by adopting diets that are high in carbs, sugar, and bad fats. I can't really solve this problem here, but I want us to be aware of it. Meal planning and diets must take cultural food differences to heart, but they don't.

Take me, for example. I'm 100 percent Italian. In my big Italian family, eating is a huge focus of daily life and get-togethers. We have full-course meals with lots and lots of pasta. So, going on a keto or low-carb diet all the time just would not work for me, culturally.

People should not have to turn their back on their ethnic favorites. Any meal plan worth its salt should incorporate foods from different cultures.

4. Meal plans don't account for food intolerances.

Meal plans often call for foods to which many people are highly sensitive. The top offenders are egg whites, dairy, gluten, soy, corn, peanuts, added sugar, or alcohol. So, following a meal plan that includes foods to which you react can be highly uncomfortable or even unhealthy.

For perspective, there are two types of food sensitivities: food intolerances and food allergies. A food allergy is a strong immune reaction due to certain foods. You eat something and an allergic reaction erupts, manifesting as hives, itching, or eczema; swelling of your lips, face, tongue, and throat, or other parts of the body; wheezing, nasal congestion, or trouble breathing, among other symptoms.

A food intolerance is much sneakier. It is a mild inflammatory chemical reaction whereby a body is unable to digest some types of food. Its symptoms can be more subtle: gas, cramps, bloating; heartburn; headaches; irritability or nervousness. Food intolerances can also cause cravings, make you feel generally unwell, and complicate your efforts to eat in a healthy way.

You simply can't follow a blanket meal plan if you suffer food sensitivities, or even suspect that you might. In fact, you need to follow an "elimination diet," in which you refrain from eating certain foods for a period of time to see how you feel. See page 233 for more about this.

Let me add that meal plans typically emphasize eating the same foods over and over. Unfortunately, this kind of repetitive eating increases the odds of immune responses, such as food intolerances. Vary your food choices.

5. Meal plans don't teach you anything about your individual nutritional needs.

Nutrition is highly individualized, and your nutritional requirements change over time. What your body needed at age twenty-five is a lot different from what you need at age fifty-five, due to fluctuating hormones, level of physical activity, and other changes.

For the most part, unless you do resistance training, you can't eat the same number of calories each day as you did when you were younger, or else you could easily gain extra fat, especially around your belly. Older adults require even higher levels of some nutrients compared to younger people. Nutrients that become especially important as you age include protein, vitamin D, calcium, and vitamin B_{12}. One study followed 2,066 elderly people over three years. It found those

AN ELIMINATION DIET IN FIVE EASY STEPS

Step 1: Write down in your journal what you eat daily, or refer to the two-week tracking data you put together from the previous chapter.

Step 2: Note any symptoms that crop up after a meal: gas, bloating, tummy aches, constipation, headaches, skin flare-ups, poor sleep, and so forth. Dairy products, such as cheese and milk, along with wheat, yeast, legumes, nuts, and eggs, and a lot of everyday foods that include even small amounts of these ingredients, are on the list of foods that can make you feel unwell.

Step 3: Eliminate one food to remove from your diet and see how you feel for two weeks. Let's say that every time after eating bread, you notice get headaches. It's best to eliminate that one offending food. Don't try to eliminate several foods at once, or else you'll never figure out which one is making you ill. If that food is a culprit for your symptom, expect to probably feel better in a few days. But give it at least two weeks.

Step 4. If you notice nothing, then move on to the next food and see how you feel. And if it isn't a problem—that's okay. Just keep monitoring and repeating the process until you start to get an idea as to which food or foods are triggering your symptoms.

Step 5. Later, reintroduce the foods, one at a time, in small amounts. Again, don't reintroduce more than one type of offender at the same time, or you won't know which of them might be negatively affecting you. If you notice that you become symptomatic when you eat them, it's best to eliminate them altogether.

who ate the most protein daily lost 40 percent *less* muscle mass than people who ate the least.

Meal plans are just too generic and not focused on what the body truly needs during various life stages, so you miss your big chance to learn how to make healthier, more enjoyable, more *lasting, and real* changes. Everyone is different when it comes to their path to health and what works for them and their lifestyle.

WHAT IF THERE WAS A BETTER WAY?

There is. Above all, you are your own best meal planner. All the tools you need are within you; you just might require a bit of guidance and education to bring them out. For long-term success, let me suggest alternative strategies to help you plan your meals intuitively, overcome bad eating habits, and design a way of eating based on your individual preferences.

Train the Behavior, Not the Solution

For long-term success, you may have to take some baby steps at first. Look at your diet and your eating habits as they stand right now.

Do you eat several fast-food cheeseburgers through the week?

Are you getting enough fiber from whole grains and other high-fiber foods each week?

Do you typically shun vegetables?

If you answered yes to any of these questions, the solution, of course, is to stop eating cheeseburgers, eat more fiber, and start piling a few more veggies on your plate. But starting with the solution isn't the answer.

You've got to first "train the behavior" to change less-than-desirable eating habits so that they practically disappear from your life.

How do you do that?

Pick one bad eating habit to work on. Let's say, you don't eat enough vegetables. Set a nutrition goal to eat a bowl of vegetables a day. Implement that change and only that change. Then, as I explained in Chapter 10, connect vegetable eating with the positive signals your body is now sending you. Realize that eating vegetables makes you feel better and look better.

You've now trained yourself to eat more vegetables. You've trained the behavior.

If there is another behavior you need to train, move on to that one next. Taking small, realistic changes leads to healthy behaviors that eventually become second nature.

Another option that works well if you aren't ready to limit or eliminate certain foods is to simply *add* a healthy food option. For example, instead of cutting out or reducing soda intake, you can just increase water intake. Oftentimes, the positive feelings lead to healthy behaviors.

Put Up Barriers Between Yourself and a Bad Eating Habit

Your environment influences your habits, good or bad. So, the best way to improve your habits is to change your environment, which generally includes places and people. Using the example of smoking: Suppose you're a smoker. If you hang out with smokers, for instance, then you are much more likely to continue your smoking habit. But if you surround yourself with healthy, nonsmoking friends, you're in a better position to adopt their healthy habits.

Let's move this discussion to food. Rather than having junk food easily accessible in your home and fighting with yourself to not eat it, try not having it in your home at all in the first place. Then, if you do get a strong craving for junk food, rather than going through the process of fighting your urges, allow yourself to have a single serving of junk food as long as you drive to the store and get it. This barrier tends to slow us down and gives us enough time to pause and become aware of our behavior. "Do I really want a single cookie bad enough to drive to the store?" Probably not!

So, to build and cement healthy eating habits, your environment must be set up for success.

Identify Your Favorite Healthy Foods

The next step is to ask yourself which macro foods you like. What are your favorite fats? Proteins? Carbs? Take into consideration your cultural and ethnic preferences.

If you're coming from a period of rigid meal plans and feel that you don't even know what foods you prefer because you've just been forcing yourself to eat what's on that plan, do some experimenting. Try out some different foods and recipes and see whether you like them. Make a list of your favorites—foods that satisfy you. Plan your meals around them.

Balance Your Meals

Most meals are structured with a protein, fat, and carbohydrate, both starchy and nonstarchy. If you have these macros at each meal, chances are that you'll intuitively meet your calorie and macro requirements each day.

I recommend that you plan each meal to include a low-calorie, high-fiber vegetable; a protein and fat; and a starchy complex carbohydrate, such as a root vegetable, a starchy vegetable, a fruit (only one a day), or a grain. (Use the lists on pages 209, 211–212, and 215–216 to guide you.) Follow this formula for creating meals; it's really the crux of what you need to know.

Sequence Your Meals

This is a superimportant habit to adopt. As you sit down to the table, eat your foods in the following order:

1. Low-calorie, high-fiber vegetable
2. Protein and fat
3. Starchy carbohydrate

Eating in this sequence increases satiety because veggies, protein, and fat are the most filling. Once you get to your carb, you may not eat all of it, curtailing your carb intake. Also, if you start with your carb, you tend to eat too fast and possibly overeat. What's more, proteins and fats are essential for health, whereas carbs are not, so it makes sense to prioritize them first and eat carbs last.

Minimize Snacking

As for snacks, I don't believe we need them. They provide unnecessary extra calories that could be reserved for your main meals. But if you like snacks, I suggest that they be whole, natural foods—nothing processed—packaged in caloric proportioned servings, such as 100 calories of nuts put in a snack bag, or a single piece of fresh fruit or a hard-boiled egg.

When you feel hungry between meals, it could simply be a sign that you need some water. Drink a couple of glasses of water and wait for half an hour to see whether getting a drink eliminates the hunger pangs. You may be able to save yourself from unnecessary calories from snacks by staying well hydrated with water.

NUTRITIONAL GUIDELINES FOR SUCCESS

1. Drink mostly water. There are hardly any situations in which "drinking your calories"—such as in commercial juices, sodas, or other beverages—is a good idea. Black coffee and tea are perfectly healthy for most people too.
2. Listen to your thirst. It is an excellent gauge for water consumption. If you're unsure of how much water to drink daily, a good, but not set-in-stone rule is that light-colored urine signifies that you are well hydrated. A dark yellow typically means you need more water; very clear urine means you might be drinking too much water.
3. Eat more unprocessed foods, such as whole fruits, vegetables, nuts, seeds, organically raised meats, fish, poultry, eggs, and so forth, and fewer processed foods.
4. Aim for foods made with one to four ingredients. They are the "cleanest" and generally the best for maintaining your health.
5. Organic, minimally processed, well-sourced dairy may be very healthy, depending on the individual, but may be unhealthy or reactive for others.

---

continues

continued

6. Use saturated fat, minimally processed oils for high-temperature cooking, sautéing, and frying. They are the least likely to be damaged by high temperatures. At high temperatures, unstable oils (including many vegetable oils) tend to be inflammatory to the body.

7. Avoid heavily processed oils, such as canola, corn, soy, and safflower. These tend to be high in omega-6 fatty acids. Consuming too many of these fatty acids can trigger inflammation in the body.

8. Avoid foods that contain additives, preservatives, pesticides, colorings, artificial sweeteners, and other chemicals. These compounds offer little to no health benefits (in some cases they are unhealthy) and are added primarily to dramatically increase the palatability of food. These ingredients make heavily processed foods so powerful at promoting overeating. Avoiding foods with these ingredients will help you eat an appropriate amount for good health.

9. Eat until you are satisfied, but not until you are full. You should not feel "stuffed" or bogged down. Imagine being totally full is at 100 percent, then eat until you feel only 75 percent full. Also, you should feel as if you can engage in a moderately intensive activity right after your meal, without any issues.

10. Vary your food choices. Explore new recipes, cuisines, or cooking techniques.

11. Do not be afraid of eating fat. It is an essential macronutrient.

12. Don't limit sodium unless otherwise specified by your doctor. Previous claims on the dangers of sodium were based on poor studies and have since been rebutted. Use mineral-rich pink Himalayan salt or well-sourced sea salt. If you're avoiding heavily processed food, you've automatically cut back on sodium because those foods are highly laced with salt.

13. Eat as many or as few meals as works best for your body. Most people find two meals a day are ideal.

14. Make small changes and improvements to what you *already normally eat and enjoy*, one small step at a time.

RAW FITNESS TRUTH #9

CHEAT MEALS STALL YOUR MOMENTUM.

More often than not, I hear what seems like far too many people getting excited for their "cheat day" . . . which usually falls on a Saturday . . . when there's a big event . . . and all the worst foods.

I also hear many variations—cheat day, cheat meal, refeed, etc. It's time to make some sense of it all.

Let's start with the fact that today's focus is cheat *meal*. *Not* day. There is no reason to dedicate an *entire* day to eating crap, convincing yourself you deserve it, when really it just hurts your progress.

Honestly, I'm not a big fan of cheat meals, unless you are super-lean and in supermuscular shape—and have been that way for a long time. For the rest of us, cheat meals block momentum, provoke guilt, and maintain a poor relationship with food.

If you are over 15 percent body fat and just starting a diet, having a cheat meal is a very bad idea. I don't care if it's Sunday football and there's nachos and beer. When you're holding on to extra fat, it's more likely you will store that cheat meal as more fat.

Okay. Suppose you indulge in something high calorie. I get it. We're human. We may all have a moment (keyword: moment, not weeks and months) of weakness where we slip up. If that happens by accident, don't let it throw you off. Just get back on the wagon and see it as a lesson learned.

There is nothing wrong with eating something that is unhealthy. In fact, as I explained earlier, doing so can be healthy when part of a celebration or bonding with family. In those cases, it is a different part of your well-being. When you give yourself permission to enjoy a favorite food every now and then, you've created balance in your diet and your life.

The idea of a cheat day or meal is the opposite of balance. The name says it all: *cheat*. Cheating means naughty. When you cheat on a test, you're a bad student. When you cheat on your partner,

continues

continued

you're a dishonest, hurtful mate. And when you cheat on your diet, you let your body down. In almost every case, cheating makes you feel guilty, stressed, anxious, discouraged, and completely down on yourself. It encourages unhealthy behaviors around food and an unhealthy relationship with food (see next section).

I believe in making your overall eating experience count. Enjoy satisfying and nourishing foods and what they're doing to your body. If you can enjoy some pizza or cookies with a loved one, more power to you. Savor all your meals in an aware state with gratefulness. Then it is not cheating. It is healthy, balanced eating.

Work on your relationship with food

The thoughts you have related to food and your ability to lose weight will have a direct impact on how quickly (or if) you lose weight. Work on making small mental shifts in your relationship with food each day. One way you can do this is by noticing how you feel when you start to eat something that does not fit with your goals. Then, you can make the connection between how you were feeling and what you ate. Do you go to junk food when you are feeling tired? If you realize that this is a pattern, you can start looking for other ways to deal with your fatigue that do not include eating junk food. A quick walk outside can provide a similar boost in energy and will not sabotage your weight loss efforts. Small changes like this will eventually add up to a much healthier life.

There will always be hundreds, probably thousands of diets, products, and procedures out there, promising to get you in shape fast. It's a sixty-billion-dollar industry, after all, with no signs of slowing down. But keep in mind that most don't work. Indeed, about 80 percent of Americans are unable to lose weight effectively and keep it off with dieting, says the *American Journal of Clinical Nutrition*.

Fortunately, intuitive eating shows us that the key to success is to enjoy healthy food that fits your lifestyle, culture, and doesn't leave you feeling guilty or hungry.

When you're ready to become an intuitive eater and make these changes—and I know you are—hit the button and say, "This is it!"

THE RESISTANCE TRAINING REVOLUTION LIFESTYLE

"I want to live to be one hundred!"

How often have you heard someone say this? Have you said it yourself? I sure have.

So—a life at one hundred? Is it possible?

Yes. In the past, however, scientists felt that the human life span had reached its limit. But recently, several studies have refuted this claim. In an analysis of Japanese women, who make up a growing number of centenarians, or people over age one hundred, researchers at the Netherlands Interdisciplinary Demographic Institute analyzed aging trends and suggested that the maximum human life span may increase to 125 years by 2070. In rare cases, this is already happening. The longest documented human life was that of Jeanne Calment, a Frenchwoman who died at age 122.

And scientists at McGill University in Montreal similarly found no evidence that maximum human life span has stopped increasing. By analyzing trends in the life spans of the longest-living individuals from the United States, the United Kingdom, France, and Japan for each year since 1968, they revealed that both maximum and average life spans may continue to increase far into the foreseeable future.

We already know from historical statistics that life expectancy has been increasing for a long time. In 1900, it was around 46 to 48 years. Between 1980 and 2010, life expectancy increased from 70 to 76 years for men and from 77 to 81 years for women, according to the Centers for Disease Control (CDC).

When I think about living to age one hundred, I know this: It is really important for me to live healthy *today and every day*, so that as I approach the centenarian mark, I will be independent, free of major health issues, active, able to move my own furniture, pay my own bills, and still take care of my loved ones—all with a sense of purpose, day in and day out.

So, what about a healthy life at one hundred? Is it possible? Yes. I've seen it firsthand. Later in my personal training career, I specialized in training older adults. There was Caroline, for example, whom I trained for fourteen years, once a week, well into her eighties. She had always prioritized her health. She was a vibrant fireball, enjoying life, socializing, and having fun dating men she met on a dating app.

James was another client—an active guy who swam and rode his bike daily, even in the rain. I remember when he came to me at age sixty-nine, wondering whether he should get his hormones tested. I gave him a thumbs-up. It turned out that his testosterone levels were that of a twenty-year-old, and he wasn't even taking testosterone!

In addition to these amazing clients, a hero of mine was always Jack LaLanne. I saw him one time at a big fitness expo. After he came out onstage, the audience would not stop their cheering and clapping so that he could speak. So, he got down on the floor and started doing one-arm push-ups. I think he was in his seventies at the time.

All of these are testimony to the benefits resistance training and an active lifestyle have on our older population—and how they keep you young.

All good news! Growing old—and doing it in a healthy, fit, active manner sure beats the alternative.

This is all a part of living better, not just living longer. Living better means being mobile, being independent, and enjoying great health.

So, what can you do today, no matter your age, to ensure that you thrive in your life, as opposed to surviving on medicines, machines, or hip or knee replacements?

I scoured the scientific literature to find the answers. What emerged are five key Resistance Training Revolution lifestyle actions you can take now to almost guarantee a golden age of vigorous, active, independent, and disease-free living.

FIVE STEPS TO LIVING WELL AND LIVING LONG

1. Stay strong.

Physical strength is an excellent predictor of longevity. The stronger you are, the more likely you are to live longer. The opposite is also true, with physical weakness being an accurate predictor of early death.

The fact that people with low muscle strength don't typically live as long as their stronger peers was revealed in a recent, fascinating study.

After adjusting for sociodemographic factors, chronic health conditions, and smoking history, researchers found that people with low muscle strength are 50 percent more likely to die earlier.

The study measured hand grip strength. For the study, which appears in the *Journal of Gerontology: Medical Sciences*, researchers analyzed data from a nationally representative sample of 8,326 men and women, ages sixty-five and older, who were part of the University of Michigan's Health and Retirement Study.

Grip strength can be measured using a device called a dynamometer, which a patient squeezes to measure their strength in kilograms. Researchers identified muscle weakness as having a hand grip strength less than 39 kg for men and 22 kg for women.

Based on the data, 46 percent of the sample population was considered weak at baseline. By comparison, only 10 to 13 percent were considered weak using other cut-points derived from less representative samples.

Prioritize your strength-building strategy, regardless of your age. Strength not only keeps you young, it also improves balance—a superimportant factor as you get older. Without good balance, you're prone to falls and bone breakage, which can land you in the hospital and possibly lead to permanent disability. You must have a strong body to have an able body.

As I've pointed out previously, longevity-based resistance training requires only two days a week of working out to stay youthful throughout your life.

2. Move!

Beyond resistance training at least twice a week, you can escape ill health and disability by simply moving your body throughout the day. In my opinion, the best way to do that is to walk, bike, hike, or swim, to name just a few daily and beneficial activities.

Do anything but sit! If you spend most of each workday sitting at your desk, your fingers the only part of your body moving with any intensity, you might be in trouble. Technology allows us to work from the relative comfort of our desk, without having to break a sweat or even stand up. Once the workday is over, we transition straight from desk to car to couch, taking barely a step in between.

The ease of our modern workday could come at the expense of our longevity. A study of older women in the *American Journal of Preventive Medicine* found that sitting for long stretches of time increases the odds of an untimely death. The more hours women in the study spent sitting at work, driving, lying on the couch watching TV, or engaged in other leisurely pursuits, the greater their odds of dying early from all causes, including heart disease and cancer.

And here's the kicker: even women who exercised regularly risked shortening their life span if most of their daily hours were sedentary ones.

How exactly sitting contributes to reduced longevity isn't clear, but there are a few possible mechanisms. Couch-potato behavior has been linked to an increased risk of the development of chronic conditions, such as type 2 diabetes and cardiovascular disease. Plus, when you sit, you burn fewer calories than you would while standing, and you demand little effort from your muscles. Sitting too much can also lead to other behaviors that contribute to obesity and heart disease, such as watching TV while snacking on processed snack food.

At the very least, make walking your "movement practice." And do it briskly. One study found that overweight people who walked at a brisk pace lived fifteen to twenty years longer than those who walked more slowly.

There's a walking strategy that I used to think was bogus: parking farther away from stores in parking lots to increase your walking distance. But then studies came out showing that this technique added two to three thousand steps to your day automatically!

Another suggestion: Try walking fifteen minutes after each of your main meals. This logs a full forty-five minutes of walking into your day. Walk and you're stimulating blood and oxygen circulation, improving your digestion, and counteracting the danger of too much sitting. Adopting a movement practice is so easy and definitely improves your longevity.

3. Avoid processed foods.

Do you want to get old fast?

I'm sure your answer is a loud "No *way!*"

Then, don't eat processed foods. These foods, which I covered earlier, create chronic inflammation in the body, and most adults over the age of thirty-five already have this going on. It unleashes its fury when pro-inflammatory substances continue to be released into your body over time, attacking your healthy cells, blood vessels, and tissues instead of protecting them.

Unhealthy cells, vessels, and tissues *equal* premature aging—skin that increasingly looks older than it should, bones that get weaker than they should, depleted energy, and a brain that gets increasingly cloudy too. Processed foods are loaded with pro-inflammatory ingredients that fuel this rapid-aging chain of events.

Is there an "antiaging diet," then? Well, science does have some definitive answers based on studying the longest-lived populations in the world—areas referred to as Blue Zones by author and researcher Dan Buettner. In his book called *The Blue Zones*, Buettner described five known Blue Zones:

Icaria (Greece), an island where people eat a Mediterranean diet rich in fish, olive oil, red wine, and home grown vegetables.

Ogliastra, Sardinia (Italy), home to some of the oldest men in the world. They live in mountainous regions where they typically work on farms and eat lots of natural foods harvested from the land.

Okinawa (Japan), home to the world's oldest women, who eat a lot of vegetables and soy-based foods.

Nicoya Peninsula (Costa Rica), where the diet is based around beans and corn tortillas.

The Seventh-Day Adventists in Loma Linda, California, a very religious group of people. They're strict vegetarians and live in tight-knit communities.

All these diets are different, but they have two things in common. First, they are centered on natural, whole foods—nothing processed. This means that Blue Zone folks are taking in nutrients used for energy, health, and antiaging.

Second, none of the people in Blue Zones overeats—which may be a very important antiaging strategy. In fact, at three research centers, a study funded by the National Institutes of Health looked into the value of calorie control to fight aging. The ongoing CALERIE Study (Comprehensive Assessment of Long-Term Effects of Reducing Intake of Energy) is showing that we can live longer, age more slowly, and be more resistant to disease by sustained calorie restriction as long as we eat sufficient amounts of nonprocessed, nutrient-rich food.

Bottom line: These are principles endorsed by the Resistance Training Revolution lifestyle. Eat whole foods, an intuitive diet, and limit, or, if possible, eliminate, heavily processed food.

What you eat matters for your overall health and longevity. Get your calories from foods that are nourishing and real. Limit your intake of heavily processed foods—and don't go overboard on calories.

4. Stay connected.

Many lives are cut short due to factors not related to resistance training, physical activity, and diet. One of these factors is social isolation. Researchers have found that it reduces average longevity more than twice as much as heavy drinking and more than three times as much as obesity (which is often a consequence of loneliness and isolation). Further, loneliness is as physically dangerous as smoking fifteen cigarettes a day and contributes to cognitive decline, including a more rapid advance of Alzheimer's disease.

For a long, happy, and productive life, invest in your relationships. Stay in touch with family, participate in clubs, organizations, and social events; volunteer; and be a part of a community of people who surround you.

Just do not isolate! People who stay connected with family, community, and friends live longer than those who are isolated.

I know I'm a better person because of my family and my Mind Pump partners. They give me support, feedback about health, and overall advice. I lean on them, and it makes a huge difference in my life.

5. Maintain a spiritual practice.

A spiritual practice—whether it is going to church, participating in a meditation group, enjoying nature, or connecting to a higher being through prayer—gives your life a sense of purpose, helps you contemplate big questions about life's meaning, and helps you apply these qualities to your challenging circumstances in your life.

Studies overwhelmingly show spiritual or religious correlations to better health and well-being. I came across a 2014 article in *Religions* that reviewed hundreds of studies, reporting that people with a spiritual life have less depression, suicide, alcohol and drug use, and greater happiness, meaning, purpose, hope, and optimism than do people without any spiritual practice. Also, having a spiritual practice has been shown to boost physical health in terms of better immunity, better endocrine and cardiovascular health, and less risk of heart disease and cancer, and lower blood pressure—and greater longevity by seven years!

I've also learned that people with a spiritual practice have a stronger will to live. I've trained a lot of doctors and surgeons over the course of my career. I'd always ask them: If someone loses his or her will to live, what is their prognosis? They'd all tell me: once the will to live is gone, they pass away pretty quickly.

A spiritual practice is an essential tool in promoting longevity, but more important, it helps us answer life's big questions—what is the point of my life? Am I making contributions? Is my life meaningful—while giving us hope in the face of serious illnesses and meeting the challenges of loss and disappointment that life tosses our way.

So—living to 100 or 120? Yes, it is within the realm of possibility if you take charge now. We do not have to get sick or more disabled as we get older. The healthier we are now, the healthier we will be in our older years—and, quite possibly, we will protect ourselves from life-threatening diseases, such as cancer and Alzheimer's disease.

Stay strong and active, nutritionally healthy, connected to community, and involved in a spiritual practice. These help us live longer and better while getting older.

Old age doesn't have to be what it used to be. Thank goodness!

CHECK YOUR SUCCESS

This is the end of the book. But it is the beginning and the continuation of an empowering journey for you. Along the way, I encourage you to keep track of your progress, as you enjoy greater energy, renewed health and strength, muscle development and the contours that come with it, and more time, control, and freedom in every area of your life.

Monitoring and tracking your progress isn't some obsessive or self-absorbed activity. It is a way to reinforce yourself in a positive way. It helps sustain your momentum.

Every three weeks, go back to Chapter 3—Forgotten Factors for a Great Body—and retake the tests and questionnaires.

How's your posture now?
Your pain level?
Shoulder mobility?
Lower body strength?
Core strength?
Your waist-to-hip ratio?

On a broader note, what about your overall strength? Are you reaching for heavier resistance from week to week? As a general rule, because your workouts include overload (meaning you've challenged your muscles to work harder over time, by increasing resistance), you should be able to move weights or other resistance that is up to 10 percent heavier—or hold such moves as planks for longer—after every two weeks or so.

Or how do you look in the mirror? If you want visual evidence of how your body is changing, consider checking your reflection. Like what you see? I hope so.

How do your clothes feel? This is a good gauge for most people. But don't expect your clothes to become looser necessarily; you may actually fill them out a bit better. This can happen because you're putting on muscle.

It's okay to weigh yourself on the scale periodically too. Having numbers to check can help you stay the course. Many different studies of "successful losers" have shown, time and time again, that people who step on the scale regularly tend to keep their weight off over the long term.

So, how often should you weigh in? Once a week at most, I feel. That's my usual recommendation because weight fluctuates so much. Any more than that and you can become frustrated if you don't see progress.

Remember too that resistance training progress isn't always linear. Other positive clues like having more energy for workouts, quality sleep, A-plus annual checkups, and better flexibility and mobility are valuable indicators too.

How's your diet? Once you've become an intuitive eater, your hankerings for sugar and processed foods should mellow out (and may even go away completely). If you load up on lean proteins, plant foods, and healthy fats with every meal, you will find that eventually you won't want the junk.

Your gut will thank you too. Retake the following gut assessment test and congratulate yourself for improvements.

GUT ASSESSMENT

To Test:

Read the following statements and answer yes or no to each.

1. I experience frequent diarrhea (more than once a week).
   Yes or No

2. I experience frequent constipation (less than one stool movement a day more than once a week).
   Yes or No

3. My stomach frequently aches after I eat.
   Yes or No

4. I frequently feel bloated after a meal.
   Yes or No

5. I experience excessive belching.
   Yes or No

6. I experience excessive foul flatulence (gas).
   Yes or No

7. I suffer from frequent heartburn (sharp, burning, or like a tightening sensation in the chest, often a few hours after a meal).
   Yes or No

8. I feel groggy after eating.
   Yes or No

9. I have more than one food sensitivity (foods that upset my digestive system).
   Yes or No

Scoring

If you answered yes to more than three statements, you may have gut issues that might need to be addressed by a health-care practitioner—although I'm sure you have improved. If not, continue to follow an elimination diet, or see a specialist to help.

After regular resistance training, you may require more clean food to keep burning calories and fuel your workouts. Keep tabs on this through tracking. If you do notice you're eating more since you've started crushing your workouts, that's okay. Just make sure you're adding real, whole foods.

Beyond these physical parameters, think about your lifestyle. Perhaps you've never felt more rested. Resistance training not only boosts your daytime energy but your sleep quality too. When you get on a regular resistance training schedule, expect to sleep more soundly and deeply than before you started. Retake the following sleep assessment.

SLEEP ASSESSMENT

To Test:

Read the following statements and answer yes or no to each.

1. **I find it difficult to fall asleep at bedtime.**
   Yes or No
2. **I usually don't remember my dreams.**
   Yes or No
3. **I wake up feeling stiff and achy.**
   Yes or No
4. **After waking up, I do not feel rested.**
   Yes or No
5. **I wake up earlier in the morning than I would like to.**
   Yes or No
6. **I am often sleepy and groggy throughout the day.**
   Yes or No
7. **I often wake up in the middle of the night.**
   Yes or No
8. **My mind races at night, preventing me from falling asleep.**
   Yes or No

Scoring

Congratulate yourself on improvements! Change up your sleep game if you still need to improve the quality of your sleep.

How's your stress level? It may help you resist excessive worry and anxiety too. Several small studies have found reductions in anxiety when resistance training is done regularly for six weeks or longer. Retake the following stress assessment.

STRESS ASSESSMENT

To Test:

Read the following statements and answer yes or no to each.

1. **I rarely get angry or tense because of things that are outside my control.**
   Yes or No
2. **I rarely feel nervous and tense.**
   Yes or No
3. **I can cope with all the things I have to do.**
   Yes or No
4. **I rarely experience such symptoms as headaches, fatigue, tense muscles, difficulty falling asleep, or bouts of anger and hostility.**
   True or False
5. **I feel that I'm on top of things.**
   True or False
6. **I have a loving, satisfying relationship with my spouse or partner.**
   True or False
7. **I feel my life has purpose.**
   True or False

8. I am connected to a spiritual community, or I have a strong social network.
   True or False

9. I create calmness in my life through the power of prayer or meditation.
   True or False

10. I have a daily practice of gratitude.
    True or False

11. I exercise at least three or four times a week.
    True or False

12. I do not abuse alcohol or drugs.
    True or False

13. If things aren't going well, I tend to view the situation as temporary rather than permanent.
    True or False

14. If I do get stressed, I can change my thinking to calm down.
    True or False

Scoring

Less stressed than before? I hope so! Keep engaging in stress-reducing activities such as working out, meditating, prayer, going on long walks, and taking time away from work and obligations to relax. Recognize the source of your stress and take steps to mitigate it.

Think about your relationships too. How have they been impacted by your resistance training lifestyle? I've seen couples who train together transform their relationships by encouraging each other and letting go of their stresses and tensions. They rediscover their youthful selves by achieving a more attractive body; greater strength, mobility, and flexibility; confidence; and of course, better performance in the bedroom. Working out is the new making out!

I'm not kidding. Exercise increases the levels of oxytocin. This is the "love hormone" associated with romance, empathy, trust, and relationship building.

As for your kids, you'll now be an example for them—by working out and behaving as you would want them to do. You are the model of possibility for them. Lead that way, and your children will follow.

All these powerful payoffs result from taking it just one step at a time. If I ever had to climb a really high mountain, I would absolutely shut down if I looked up too far. I might glance up occasionally to take in the hike ahead, but my attention would have to be fixed on where my feet were going next, or I'd stumble and fall. I'd have to take things one step at a time, one muscle ache at a time, one breath at a time. And that's what you have to do on this journey.

Enjoy every step now, embracing your full strength, energy, vitality, and the elevated performance and success that follow. Being a part of the Resistance Training Revolution to reboot your metabolism and recharge your mind, body, and life is, hands down, the best investment you will ever make in your success.

The mountaintop awaits you, my friend!

ACKNOWLEDGMENTS

This book was brought to life because of an amazing team of people:

My Mind Pump Media business partners and close friends Doug Egge, Adam Schafer, and Justin Andrews. I'm grateful for their support and friendship.

My wife, Jessica, for her unwavering support and for being my biggest fan.

Catrina Garcia, for keeping me organized and on task (which can be an almost impossible task).

My parents, Domenico and Josephine, for always encouraging me to follow my dreams and for risking everything to come to this country to create a good life for me and my siblings.

Rick Broadhead, my agent, who led me through the entire process of turning an idea into a book.

Dan Ambrosia, Cisca Schreefel, and the entire team at Hachette Book Group for believing in me and seeing that it is indeed time for this revolution.

And Maggie Greenwood-Robinson, for putting all my thoughts, ideas, and concepts into words for this project.

RESOURCES

Resistancetrainingrevolution.com for video demonstrations of the exercises in the workouts coached by Sal

Mapsmacro.com for a macronutrient and calorie calculator to help you figure out how much to eat for your body and goals

Mindpumpfree.com for free fitness guides

REFERENCES

INTRODUCTION

J. A. Bennie et al., "Muscle-Strengthening Exercise Among 397,423 U.S. Adults: Prevalence, Correlates, and Associations with Health Conditions," *American Journal of Preventive Medicine* 55 (2018): 864–874.

CHAPTER 1: THE CARDIO CRAZE: WHY IT'S MAKING YOU FAT

Kevin D. Hall et al., "Ultra-Processed Diets Cause Excess Calorie Intake and Weight Gain: An Inpatient Randomized Controlled Trial of *Ad Libitum* Food Intake," *Clinical and Translational Report* 30 (2019): 67–77.

D. R. Laddu et al., "25-Year Physical Activity Trajectories and Development of Subclinical Coronary Artery Disease as Measured by Coronary Artery Calcium: The Coronary Artery Risk Development in Young Adults (CARDIA) Study," *Mayo Clinic Proceedings* 92 (2017): 1660–1670.

H. Pontzer et al., "Hunter-Gatherers as Models in Public Health," *Obesity Reviews* 19, suppl. 1 (2018): 24–35.

P. Schnohr et al., "Dose of Jogging and Long-Term Mortality: The Copenhagen City Heart Study," *Journal of the American College of Cardiology* 65 (2015): 411–419.

J. Treasure and L. Eid, "Eating Disorder Animal Model," *Current Opinion in Psychiatry* 32 (2019): 471–477.

CHAPTER 2: DO WHAT YOU'RE NOT DOING TO BURN FAT

J. R. Alley et al., "Effects of Resistance Exercise Timing on Sleep Architecture and Nocturnal Blood Pressure," *Journal of Strength and Conditioning Research* 29 (2015): 1378–1385.

J. A. Blumenthal et al., "Is Exercise a Viable Treatment for Depression?" *ACSM's Health & Fitness Journal* 16 (2012): 14–21.

K. M. Broadhouse et al., "Hippocampal Plasticity Underpins Long-Term Cognitive Gains from Resistance Exercise in MCI," *Neuroimage: Clinical*, Epub January 14, 2020.

E. Cava et al., "Preserving Healthy Muscle During Weight Loss," *Advances in Nutrition* 8 (2017): 511–519.

S. R. Collier et al., "Changes in Arterial Distensibility and Flow-Mediated Dilation After Acute Resistance vs. Aerobic Exercise," *Journal of Strength and Conditioning Research* 24 (2010): 2846–2852.

A. Cuevas-Sierra et al., "Diet, Gut Microbiota, and Obesity: Links with Host Genetics and Epigenetics and Potential Applications," *Advances in Nutrition* 10, suppl. 1 (2019): S17–S30.

K. Duchowny, "Do Nationally Representative Cutpoints for Clinical Muscle Weakness Predict Mortality? Results from 9 Years of Follow-up in the Health and Retirement Study," *Journals of Gerontology: Series A* 74 (2019): 1070–1075.

M. S. Fragala et al., "Resistance Training for Older Adults: Position Statement from the National Strength and Conditioning Association," *Journal of Strength and Conditioning Research* 33 (2019): 2019–2052.

L. M. Hornbuckle et al., "Effects of High-Intensity Interval Training on Cardiometabolic Risk in Overweight and Obese African-American Women: A Pilot Study," *Ethnic Health* 23 (2018): 752–766.

K. MacKenzie-Shalders et al., "The Effect of Exercise Interventions on Resting Metabolic Rate: A Systematic Review and Meta-analysis," *Journal of Sports Sciences* 38 (2020): 1635–1649.

R. A. Mekary et al., "Weight Training, Aerobic Physical Activities, and Long-Term Waist Circumference Change in Men," *Obesity* 23 (2015): 461–467.

S. Melov et al., "Resistance Exercise Reverses Aging in Human Skeletal Muscle," *PLoS One* 2 (2007): e465.

M. Pollock et al., "Resistance Exercise in Individuals With and Without Cardiovascular Disease," *Circulation* 10 (2000): 828–833.

C. R. Roberts et al., "Untrained Young Men Have Dysfunctional HDL Compared with Strength-Trained Men Irrespective of Body Weight," *Journal of Applied Physiology* 115 (2013): 1043–1049.

J. M. Taylor et al., "Growth Hormone Response to an Acute Bout of Resistance Exercise in Weight-Trained and Non-Weight-Trained Women," *Journal of Strength and Conditioning Research* 14 (2000): 220–227.

Y. Wang et al., "Association of Muscular Strength and Incidence of Type 2 Diabetes," *Mayo Clinic Proceedings* 94 (2019): 643–651.

C. H. Westfall, "Bone Mineral Content of Femur, Lumbar Vertebrae, and Radius in Eumenorrheic Female Athletes," master's thesis, University of Arizona, 1988.

CHAPTER 3: FORGOTTEN FACTORS FOR A GREAT BODY

National Center for Complementary and Integrative Health, "Statistics from the National Health Interview Survey, 2017," https://www.nccih.nih.gov/health/statistics-from-the-national-health-interview-survey.

M.-P. St. Onge, "Sleep-Obesity Relation: Underlying Mechanisms and Consequences for Treatment," *Obesity Reviews* 18, suppl. 1 (2017): 34–39.

X. Wanget et al., "Influence of Sleep Restriction on Weight Loss Outcomes Associated with Caloric Restriction," *Sleep* 41 (May 1, 2018).

CHAPTER 5: DO YOU REALLY WANT IT?

D. Y. Lee et al., "Appropriate Amount of Regular Exercise Is Associated with a Reduced Mortality Risk," *Medicine and Science in Sports and Exercise* 50 (2018): 2451–2458.

CHAPTER 7: THE TOTAL BODY ANYWHERE PROGRAM

B. Langton and J. King, "Utilizing Body Weight Training with Your Personal Training Clients," ACSM's *Health & Fitness Journal* 22 (2018): 44–51.

CHAPTER 8: THE TOTAL BODY DUMBBELL PROGRAM

P. A. Villablanca et al., "Nonexercise Activity Thermogenesis in Obesity Management," *Mayo Clinic Proceedings* 90 (2015): 509–519.

CHAPTER 10: THE ONLY DIET STRATEGY YOU'LL EVER NEED

J. Joo et al., "The Influence of 15-Week Exercise Training on Dietary Patterns Among Young Adults," *International Journal of Obesity* 43 (2019): 1681–1690.

CHAPTER 11: MACROS TO ACCELERATE YOUR RESULTS

M. Bagherniya et al., "The Effect of Fasting or Calorie Restriction on Autophagy Induction: A Review of the Literature," *Ageing Research Reviews* 47 (2018): 183–197.

D. K. Houston et al., "Dietary Protein Intake Is Associated with Lean Mass Change in Older, Community-Dwelling Adults: The Health, Aging, and Body Composition (Health ABC) Study," *American Journal of Clinical Nutrition* 87 (2008): 150–155.

M. A. Yunsheng, "Single-Component Versus Multicomponent Dietary Goals for the Metabolic Syndrome: A Randomized Trial," *Annals of Internal Medicine* 162 (2015): 248–257.

INDEX